Evaluating in Practice

Ian Shaw

Published by
Arena
Ashgate Publishing Limited
Gower House
Croft Road
Aldershot
Hants GU11 3HR
England

Ashgate Publishing Company
Old Post Road
Brookfield
Vermont 05036
USA

British Library Cataloguing in Publication Data

Shaw, Ian
  Evaluating in practice
  1. Social service 2. Evaluation
  I. Title
  361.3'2

Library of Congress Catalog Card Number: 95-83940

ISBN 1 85742 232 5 (hardback)
ISBN 1 85742 233 3 (paperback)

Printed and bound in Great Britain by
Hartnolls Limited, Bodmin, Cornwall

Contents

List of figures

Acknowledgements

Nick Evans, Andrew Leonard, and David and Jane Williams have alleviated the usual demands of life in ways which have made a substantial impact on this book. Thanks. Several colleagues in Cardiff and elsewhere have read and commented on various parts of the manuscript or taken on parts of my teaching while I have been writing. I am grateful in particular to Paul Atkinson, Mick Bloor, Steve Bowkett, Peter Greenhill, David Howe, Mike Maguire and Andy Pithouse.

The social workers whose views provide a crucial part of the early chapters in this book were willing to talk at length and on the record about their evaluating practices. I hope they do not feel I have too far misrepresented what they wanted to say.

Alison Shaw has been both daughter and colleague during the final stages of this book. Her contribution to the fieldwork and her comments on successive drafts of parts of this book have been greatly appreciated. Thanks.

Thanks also to those past students whose effect on this book has been greater than they remember.

Jackie Swift did the most efficient of jobs in taking off my hands the final preparation of the manuscript for the publishers.

I am grateful for copyright permission to quote from several poets, novelists and songwriters. Acknowledgements are due in particular to the following:

Curtis Brown Group Ltd for permission to quote from Margaret Atwood's novel, *The Robber Bride* published by Virago. Faber and Faber for permission to quote two extracts from the poems *Under Which Lyre* and *Numbers and Faces* by W H Auden. Reed Books for permission to quote from Malcolm Bradbury's novel, *The History Man*, published by Martin Secker and Warburg Ltd. Jonathan Cape Ltd for permission to quote extracts from the songs *Love Minus Zero/No*

Limit and *Ballad of a Thin Man* by Bob Dylan. Pan Books Ltd for permission to quote from Graham Swift's novel, *Waterland*. MacDonald and Co (Publishers) Ltd for permission to quote from Primo Levi, *The Wrench*. Sheil Land Associates Ltd for permission to quote Dannie Abse's poem, *Song for Pythagoras*, from his collection of poems *White Coat, Purple* Coat, published in 1989 by Century Hutchinson Ltd.

To Alison and Jonathan

1 Keeping social work honest

Lovers of small numbers go benignly potty,
Believe all tales are thirteen chapters long,
Have animal doubles, carry pentagrams
Are Millerites, Baconians, Flat-Earth-Men.

Lovers of big numbers go horridly mad,
Would have the Swiss abolished, all of us
Well purged, somatotyped, baptised, taught baseball:
They empty bars, spoil parties, run for Congress.

W H Auden *('Numbers and Faces')*

Is social work worth doing? And how do I know if I am doing it well, or even well enough? These questions - questions of evaluation - lie at the heart of what social work means. In this book we attempt to identify the knowledge, values and skills which are required for developing evaluation as a dimension of direct social work practice. The intention is to enable social workers, social work students and practice teachers to establish a critical, disciplined practice in partnership with service users, to evaluate their own practice, and to be rigorous in assessing the social work task.

Recent years have witnessed a rapidly expanding expectation that social work practitioners should be able to demonstrate identifiable and satisfactory outcomes from their practice. This expectation shows no signs of lessening, and is evident across a wide range of services. The reform of care in the community provisions at the beginning of the 1990s included requirements for assessment of service quality on the part of both providers and purchasers of services. The 1989 Children Act led to a major extension of assessment and planning activity by social workers, with related requirements about evaluating service process and outcomes.

Quality measures comprise a significant dimension of the work of the Social Services Inspectorate, following its increased scale and powers, and the introduction of local inspection units and complaints procedures. Principles of user satisfaction, quality management, and partnership have been deployed to assess a wide span of service objectives. Such developments require a rethinking of evaluating skills by social workers. Within the Probation Service there has also been a gradual trend towards requiring evaluation skills on the part of probation officers. These increasing expectations regarding evaluation are supported by social work education requirements, which include as part of core competencies that social workers should contribute to the maintenance, critical evaluation and development of their own professional practice, knowledge and values.

However, while these developments place steadily growing pressures on practitioners to be demonstrably accountable, none of them provides a model for evaluating as part of direct practice. Indeed, the most potent invitations to evaluate come, in the most part, from *outside* social work. Feminist writing and action, new forms of action research, the challenge to rethink the creation and control of knowledge in Third World development strategies, and above all the state of flux in the field of qualitative research methods, combine to make the development of evaluating in practice one of the most critical issues facing social work. The invitation from *within* social work stems from a mixture of management by effectiveness approaches, and the steady growth of an empirical practice movement in America. From the late 1970s American practice has been marked by an increasing pressure to base practice as much as possible on facts that are confirmed by rigorous research. Advocates of such empirical practice - now exercising a growing influence on social work in Britain - often draw parallels between research processes and treatment processes, and make the claim that basic problem solving strategies pervade both realms.

There has been an animated, even passionate, debate about the relative merits of positivist and humanist positions in social work. Our own position will be clear from this book. Yet the way in which the debate has been conducted has been in large part unhelpful. Not that there is nothing to debate. But social workers have tended to adopt entrenched positions which make it difficult to get fully inside or outside the argument. Hence, positivism becomes 'a swearword by which no-one is swearing' (Williams, 1976), and we are sometimes left with the impression that if only we were courageous enough to 'deconstruct' a problem we would be more than half way to its solution. For both positivists and committed advocates of humanist alternatives Augustine's comment is apposite - 'total abstinence is easier than perfect moderation'.

We will have cause to explore each of these potential ingredients of evaluating in practice, but our concern in this book is in large part with the spin-offs for evaluating in practice that come from recent thinking in the field of qualitative social research. Traditional arguments for ethnography, which until relatively recently proceeded roughly along the lines that qualitative methods provide a sounder portrayal of the real world than more established quantitative methods, have themselves come under sustained examination. There has been a blurring of the once firm boundary between social scientific ways of representing reality and literary forms of doing so (eg Atkinson, 1990; Denzin and Lincoln, 1994). Critics who are pessimistic about the possibility of understanding the real world, or those who want evaluation and research to take an overtly political role, both serve to re-open accepted beliefs about the relation between practice and evaluation. Some social workers have begun to explore the implications of ethnography for direct practice (eg Scott, 1989; Searight, 1988; Martin, 1995), and there are signs that some ethnographers may have a reciprocal interest in the relevance of ethnographic work for practitioner audiences (Bloor and McKeganey, 1987 and 1989; Miller and Crabtree, 1994). For example, arising out of their comparative ethnography of eight therapeutic communities, Bloor and McKeganey argue that practitioners should be among the several different audiences for ethnography. They reflect on a number of practices observed in their research which appeared to promote therapy in the settings in which they were found. Without claiming any special privilege for their conclusions, they describe those practices for practitioner audiences. We hope that a side-effect of this book will be to increase this two-way traffic.

'Sociological sadism'

Evaluation and research do not enjoy a good press among social workers. 'At best practitioners experience research as irrelevant; at worst as the process of being ripped off' (Everitt, *et al* 1992: 5). A staff member of a Home Office crime prevention project believed she was speaking for everyone when she said, 'no-one likes evaluation -

it makes us feel childlike.' This deeply felt mistrust, allied to the disempowering effects of work done by outside 'experts', lends credence to a conviction among social workers, no doubt widely held, that evaluation is alien to the core values and skills of practice. Knowing that numbers provide the rhetoric of our age, social workers often view research as an excuse for postponing painful political action, a tool to advance the career interests of academics who wish to do something they find interesting, without getting their hands or minds dirty, or as an exercise in 'datamugging' - the use of survey methods for media, commercial or political ends.   In the face of sociological generalisations and abstractions, human suffering appears to fade - the sociological sadism that Robert Merton once warned about.

Researchers have too often provided good grounds for this mistrust. Criticisms of social workers as numerically backward, or as having irrational attitudes towards counting and measuring (Philip, *et al*, 1975: xiii), serve no purpose whatever when they appeal to authorities such as Piaget or Freud in order to demean practitioners. There is, however, an odd paradox, which reveals an underlying ambivalence on the part of social workers about the value of research. Experienced practitioners exhibit a healthy scepticism of evidential claims based on the interpretation of figures or the application of research findings. Yet anecdotal impressions from long experience of teaching social research to social workers suggest that they too often regard 'lacking objectivity' as a cardinal sin.

This is not, you might think, especially relevant to our concerns in these chapters. After all, this is not a book about research, or even in any obvious sense about how to apply research for the enriching of practice. It is about what social workers do and ought to do as part of their day-to-day work. The problem, of course, is that evaluating *in* practice is inextricably tied up with evaluation *of* practice, so that attitudes to research inevitably become intertwined with attitudes to evaluating in practice. In consequence the understandable mistrust produces a weakened practice, and constitutes one reason why a book of this kind is needed. Indeed, the fact that numbers are rhetoric is no reason to duck out of evaluating what we do. Social workers are themselves involved in the practice of persuasion and claims making. Their evaluation is inevitably advocacy evaluation. Estimating the nature and scale of problems such as rape, homelessness, the involvement of young people in prostitution, or domestic violence, are works of persuasion. Persuasion is the essence of the work of groups such as Shelter, the Terence Higgins

Trust, or the Howard League.   Social workers are often sceptical of the rhetoric of others, but not always of their own or of that which stems from 'sympathetic' groups. Assuming practitioners do not want to be involved in cynical claims making, then evaluating of social workers' own rhetoric is needed (Best, 1987; 1989).   Effective persuasion requires evaluating in practice skills.

Yet it is not enough for social work academics to exhort practitioners to be more committed to evaluating in practice, given the paucity of both relevant literature and practice exemplars.   Social workers are not helped by the fact that there is almost no tradition of reflecting on and developing work on evaluating in practice.   The available relevant literature is either about providing hard pressed practitioners with user-friendly research skills (eg Edwards and Talbot, 1994), or about ways of utilising existing research to enhance and inform practice (eg Everitt *et al,* 1992). The major social work texts which follow a process model of intervention (eg Siporin, 1975; Compton and Galaway, 1989; Hepworth and Larsen, 1986; Pincus and Minahan, 1973) devote very little space to questions of evaluating, and almost always do so in the context of termination of intervention.   Standard British texts on social work practice and theory exhibit the same evaluation-blindness.   The main exception to this deficit is a fairly extensive American literature on empirical practice and specifically on methods of evaluating single cases and client systems, which works out of a positivist tradition.

We so far have highlighted two problems.   First, a weakened practice through chronic mistrust and avoidance of evaluating in practice issues, reinforced, secondly, by the failure of social work writers to reflect on and exemplify qualitative strategies of evaluating. These problems combine to diminish evaluating for and with service users. This avoidance strategy runs an even higher risk, because of the fundamental changes taking place in agency information systems. It scarcely needs saying that the advent of information technology has radical implications, opportunities and risks for social work. Information technology impinges on evaluating in practice from several directions (cf Nurius and Hudson, 1993).   Access to the Internet, electronic mail, the development of software packages that can be used in direct practice, and the gradual development of computer based learning are innovations which have special relevance to evaluating competencies.

Much of the information about evaluation trends in America summarised in Chapter Two was gained from scanning information networks, and there are numerous gopher accessible resources related to research on social work practice (Holden, Rosenberg and Weissman, 1995). The explosion in numbers of discussion lists is a specific area where social work practice has been effected. A three month monitoring of a list called SOCWORK yielded several mailings about evaluating issues. These included debate about the growing application of Geographic Information Systems (GIS) to social work and human services. GIS have potential for individual practitioners as they attempt to explore the relation between the *location* of service users and their *problems*, and in addition benefit agencies at the level of providing information about assessing service needs and project development. List subscribers were also directed to the National Association of Social Workers which markets software enabling social workers to portray individual functioning in relation to people's environment, of the kind produced by practice aids   such as genograms. The list disseminated details of the work done by the Family Development Center at Cornell University in developing the potential of computer networking for solving problems faced by social workers in the field of child abuse and neglect. SOCWORK also included useful debate during this period about whether the concept of sexual-racism adds to our understanding of sexism and racism, and an exchange covering current thinking on false memory syndrome.   Debates surrounding the relation of research and practice, and also concerning computer based learning initiatives, were present on the list in that brief period.   We recognise the problems and limitations of the information explosion, but one major advantage is that the rapid response time of discussion lists conveys the cut and thrust of debate in a way that carries an immediacy lacking in the more measured output of hard copy journals.   The growth of electronic journals is likely to further blur the edges between traditional forms of debate and on-line exchanges over the Internet.

The establishment of the Computers in Teaching Initiative (CTI) through the higher education funding councils has provided an institutionalised framework through which computer based learning gains support.   The Human Services CTI unit is based at Southampton University, and collaborative developments in pro- ducing software that can be used in social work courses offer a model which may rapidly lead on to practitioner and agency software. The 'Social Work and Information Technology' programme (Rafferty, Glastonbury, Butler and Shaw, 1995) can be searched to display a number of discussions linking information technology and evaluation. Practice software already exists, especially in the areas of welfare benefits and social work law, based on expert and semi-expert systems. An expert system is a computer programme that can be asked to give advice on the solutions to problems.

> The developer of such a system tries to incorporate the knowledge of experts in a particular field into a programme so that it is accessible and usable...In an expert system the focus shifts from data in the form of facts about cases to knowledge in the form of rules used by experts
>
> (Schuerman, 1987: 10).

Simple survey design programmes are also available (eg Questionmark), which can be utilised, with minimal training, by social workers and social work students who have no previous research knowledge.

Social workers are sensitive to the ethical and technical limitations of information technology. On one side of the debate, enthusiasts are persuaded that the World Wide Web provides channels for user access which fundamentally alters political relationships for the better. However, problems such as sexual harassment and sexual abuse through the Internet are now receiving recognition in the courts. The first generation of IT 'stake-claimers' is giving way to second generation 'settlers', with the consequence that issues about policing the Internet are receiving increasing attention. The absence of quality controls on deposits on the networks, the massive scale of information deposits, gaps in information especially from Third World countries, the continuing male-dominated nature of the information industry, and the speed of change, all create a special agenda of concerns. The use of information technology will not resolve the conflicting interests of research and social work (Steyaert, 1992). However, social work learning, practice, evaluating, and service development are all irreversibly effected by these developments. This creative tension of passion, analysis and technology lies at the heart of social work.

Doing evaluating in practice

Developments within agencies, the information explosion, and the mistrust of research and evaluation about social work are sufficient as reasons for a book on evaluating in practice. Yet they are largely external to the individual practitioner. The central justification for this book is that social work and those who receive the services provided by social workers, need the kind of practitioners that a commitment to evaluating will foster - practitioners who are able to make imaginative, lateral 'translations', who are empirically informed, who work as both outsiders and insiders within social work, who are reflexive practitioners, committed to falsifying their favourite practice, and above all are engaged to evaluate both for and with those who use their services. We have aimed to write this book around this set of commitments.

Empirically informed

There are key moments in the early stages of this book when we will step aside and listen to the stories and accounts of social workers, recently qualified social work students, and practice teachers as they reflect on their own evaluating practices. This book is not a research study, but these accounts, given for this text, provide an empirical foundation for the development of evaluating in practice competencies grounded in existing practice. The almost complete absence of previous evidence regarding practitioners' accounts of evaluating is a major part of the general neglect we referred to earlier. In reading this evidence, which provides an empirical spine to the first half of the book, much is related that can lay claim to being good practice. We will see that social workers reject, for example, the assumption that knowledge is created by outside experts and then is put into practice by social workers. Evaluating is essentially part of practice. But we will also see that evaluating is an inherently 'troublesome' ingredient of practice. It is within practice, yet at the same time different and outside. Evaluating practice is also seen as typically hard to get 'right'. Social workers recognise that evaluating practices themselves need evaluation assessment, planning and intervention.

The new data in this book need to be read from this perspective. They are the accounts which provide the essential empirical connections for developing an evaluating in practice that is not decontextualised or imposed from the outside.

'Think big, do small'

Evaluating in practice calls for 'translating' - for lateral thinking and leaps of the imagination. This is partly because of the absence of practice literature and exemplars. I beg, borrow and beachcomb through this book, and the reader is invited to do the same. But the need for imaginative leaps is also basic to doing as well as developing the kind of practice required. Qualitative research, feminist epistemologies, Third World development strategies, and other forms of action research all need translating if they are to press us into good evaluating practice. If we are to recognise and capitalise on parallels between ethnographic research and social work practice, it will call for much more than a determination to simply 'do ethnography'.

Carol Meyer suggests that, just as environmentalists say 'Think globally - act locally', so social workers should think big and do small. 'To think big and to do small is to rely on our minds' (Meyer, 1992: 299). She goes on to regret that

> One of the most serious consequences of the pragmatic policies and political philosophy of the last 10 years has been the anti-intellectualism and downgrading of the expression of independent thought.

Describing this as 'policy by popularity poll', she laments that in social work, scales, profiles, tables, graphs and surveys 'have come to substitute for hard and rigorous thinking about individuals and their situational contexts' (p302).

Much of the effort that has gone into charting the relationship between research and practice is redundant because it is about the relationship between two largely separate domains. We may recall the familiar perception test of what we perceive as foreground figure and what as background, which proceeds by asking whether we can 'see' two faces or a vase. Social workers have tended to see action and practice as 'figure' and research and understanding as 'ground'. The trick, as with the vase and the faces, is to see both as figure. This will require conceptual and methodological curiosity. Conceptual, because there is nothing so practical as a good idea, and methodological because it is no more appropriate for social workers to rely almost entirely on interviews as a way of learning about the worlds of those for whom we work, than it would be for researchers.

Outside and inside

Evaluators in practice operate at the boundaries. They are outsiders on the inside. In this respect we should not view evaluating as different from the whole of social work practice. For example, community workers' 'structural position is almost always one of interjacence, carrying out their work on the boundaries of groups and organisations in the community.' 'Lying between people...and bureaucracies' and 'in community groups but seldom, if ever, of them', community workers are located in a position which provides 'a continually testing drama' (Henderson, Jones and Thomas, 1980: 2, 3, 6). To be a marginal stranger (Thomas, 1975), who is temporarily accepted as an insider, is an inevitable and even desirable characteristic of community work practice.

Feminist critique helps at this point. There is an important feminist argument about women in social work having 'double vision' arising from being both social workers (and therefore insiders) and women (and therefore outsiders by virtue of their oppression). This double vision produces, it is argued, a 'truer' picture of the world than is possible for men. We assess the contribution of this argument on several occasions during this book, but it suffices for the present as an illustration of how translating from feminism provides a potential understanding of evaluating in practice.

It is perhaps too easy to assume that, because we work in a particular agency, we understand the nature of practice in that agency. Familiarity can obstruct the cultivation of a shared sense of puzzlement and 'anthropological strangeness' (Lofland, 1971) with colleagues and service users. As social workers we take much for granted - we operate within our 'thinking as usual' knowledge. Evaluating in practice requires that we be simultaneously an onlooker in the stalls and a member of the cast, entering as a partner with the actors (Schutz, 1971). Such evaluating in practice is ethical practice. It

> does not lead towards social engineering prescriptions based upon mathematics. It leads rather towards responsibility and integrity in one's management of changing situations of infinite complexity
>
> (Ruddock, 1981: 28).

Evaluating in practice is therefore at one and the same time both a fundamental part of practice and a critique of practice. Were the word not sadly overused, we might describe this as *critical* evaluating in practice.

Knowing and not knowing

Social workers already know much about evaluating in practice, and yet find it strange and different. The quotations at the head of each chapter are not simply literary decoration, but convey that social work is not a hermetically sealed set of professional skills and techniques, unique to the profession and with its own value base. Rather, novelists, poets and songwriters observe the world in ways which speak with relevance to evaluating in practice, and persuade us that we really do know more than we think. We will see later how Donald Schon (1983), through a detailed comparison of professional practice by an architect and a therapist, obliges us to reconsider our assumptions about the boundaries of professional ways of knowing and doing, and to recognise there is a wider community of shared knowledge about reflection on professional practices.

Yet a difficulty often experienced by social workers coming to literature about evaluation and research for the first time is the sense of not knowing the language. Even when we grasp the formal meanings of terms, the 'fringes' (the term is William James) of language are not translatable. We are soon conscious that language has secondary meanings derived from the context, and private codes derived from common past experiences. So, learning to do evaluating in practice is both simple and difficult. Simple, because we know far more than we may appreciate, and difficult because an active command of professional work is always difficult.

A skills map

This is not a handbook of evaluating in practice skills. That would need a different, fatter book. Yet practice is fundamental to the intention of the book. Rather than being a skills handbook, it is a skills *map*, an attempt at a topography, the main contours of which are outlined in the first half of the book. To change the metaphor, the general principles are followed in the later stages of the book by cartoon sketches of the kind of evaluating in practice developments that I think are both necessary and feasible.

We begin our exploration in the next chapter with an outline of evaluation developments in North America, Europe and the European Commission. The mandates for evaluation are located on these national stages, and we move on from there to describe different ways in which the relationship between understanding, investigation and action has been developed.   The relationships between knowledge and policy, understanding and action, are a central problem for evaluation at all levels.   We consider developments in applied social research, action research, practitioner research, participatory inquiry, and advocacy evaluation.

In Chapter Three we step back from the main line of argument to listen to the stories and accounts of social workers as they describe their present endeavours to evaluate in day-to-day practice.   We will discover that, whether they work in large-scale agencies or small voluntary projects, they draw a strong distinction between formal measures of evaluation within their agencies and their own self evaluation.   Each of these models of evaluation has its distinctive commitments, attitudes and activities.   Practitioners' evaluating poses several important questions which demand resolution for evaluating in practice.   We will see that social workers were preoccupied with resolving the extent to which they were personally responsible when practice went wrong.   They were also uncertain about how far explanations of cause and effect could be reached in their practice.   The perceived complexity of evidence created a constant problem in this regard.   Finally, we will see that their judgements regarding whether work had gone well or not were influenced to a major degree by the emotional rewards and penalties which social work practice entails.

If this is how practitioners seek to evaluate their practice, how does this integrate with service users' evaluations of practice?   We now know a certain amount about how service users appraise services received.   In Chapter Four we briefly review this evidence, and highlight how practitioners appear to see the relationship between their own evaluations and those of clients. We consider two significant questions.   First, is partnership in evaluating between social workers and clients likely to be straightforward or will it face special difficulties?   Second, is 'consumer satisfaction' the yardstick against which social work outcomes must be measured?

Practice occurs in specific organisational contexts, and in Chapter Five we seek to demonstrate that the culture of management and quality constrains the ways in which social workers are able to construct and test their evaluating in practice competencies.   We sketch the growth in quality management in the personal social services, and connect this to practitioners' perceptions of formal agency evaluation - 'Evaluation with a capital E', as one person described it.   Shifting relations between social work and the state together with tighter management styles have been put forward as the basis for increasing user participation in the planning, development, delivery and evaluation of community care services. We assess this argument, and also examine practitioners' views regarding the degree to which relationships with first line managers provide a culture within which evaluating in practice can flourish.

Chapters Two through to Five provide, to repeat an earlier metaphor, a topography within which evaluating in practice will be located. In Chapter Six we develop a fuller definition of evaluating in practice. This chapter is the hinge around which the book pivots. We believe that a reflexive practice, a concern with plausible evidence, a commitment to evaluate both for and with the service user, an anti-discriminatory evaluating, and an ethical purposefulness are the hallmarks of evaluating in practice. We also review the general claims of positivism in this chapter, and the inadequacies of most social work responses to the challenge posed by positivistic practice.

In Chapters Seven through to Nine we try to deliver on the claims made in the previous chapters. Following a rough and ready process model, we explore the possibilities for evaluating in practice when assessing, planning, intervening and judging outcomes. Drawing especially on qualitative research methods, we take a closer look at feminist evaluating, self-evaluation strategies, and the potential for participatory and advocacy evaluation. Social workers have relied almost exclusively on certain kinds of interviewing as the means of practice and inquiry. This has severely impoverished practice in general and evaluating in practice in particular. To begin to redress this unacceptable tradition, we explore ways in which social workers can and ought to consider *participant observation* methods together with a wider span of *interview* approaches. We advocate the 'translation' and assimilation of the various innovatory forms of *life history* and life course methods presently being developed in qualitative research. Practice records and reports are a familiar part of the genre of social work documents. Yet the potential of *practice and personal texts* for evaluating in practice has scarcely been acknowledged. We map some of these possibilities in Chapter Eight, along with an effort to recast recent interesting work on *focus groups* to exploit its potential for evaluating in practice. *Member validation* exercises, new ideas about the use of *simulated clients*, and exercises in *cultural review* are also reviewed in terms of their contribution to practice. Each of these strategies can be used to constitute and support a reflexive, falsifying, participatory and practitioner-led evaluating in practice.

A recent revival of confidence in the ability of social workers and probation officers to deliver effective interventions and achieve planned outcomes is evidence of a new belief in the potential for rehabilitative success. In Chapter Nine we will review the important claim that social work may be able to deliver an empirical practice that works, through a consideration of two of the most widely held forms in which it is made. First, we will reflect on the debate within the Probation Service about the effectiveness of treatment strategies aimed at the rehabilitation of offenders, and consider whether the negative conclusions drawn from research evaluations of probation practice in the 1960s and 1970s were born of a premature mixture of inaccuracy and pessimism. Second, we will explore the widely supported claims for the benefits of the form of practitioner research known as single-system research. We will end our consideration of evaluating in practice skills with a return to the work done on consumer satisfaction, and suggest some of the best practice inferences that can be made from this research.

This book aims to offer a provisional definition, a skills map, and a small collection of outline 'cartoons' of evaluating in practice. Doing evaluating in practice needs much more than this 'starter pack'. In particular, it must be subjected to the same evaluating through falsification, reflexive use, and participatory work with and for service users that must be demanded of social work practice as a whole.

2   The scene of the action

There are times when we have to disentangle history from fairy-tale. There are times (they come round really quite often) when good, dry, textbook history takes a plunge into the old swamps of myth and has to be retrieved with empirical fishing lines.

Graham Swift *('Waterland')*

Evaluation is on the agenda. The 1990s have been marked by a resurgent optimism about the role of evaluation in United States public policy, an expanding evaluation function in the European Commission, and a drive for programme evaluation in several European countries. Evaluation societies have emerged across national boundaries, and international organisations, including Non-Governmental Organisations working in the Third World, exercise growing evaluation functions. We open this chapter with an outline of these national, cultural and social theatres in which evaluation occurs, and locate the features of the national stage on which mandates for evaluation in social work are played out in the United Kingdom.

The relationship between knowledge and policy, understanding and action is a central problem for evaluation. The main thrust of this chapter will be to trace the attempts to square the circle of understanding, evaluation and action. Evaluating in practice, as an integral part of social work, acquires critical edge when its place is grasped within the wider scenes sketched in the following paragraphs.

Evaluation in national contexts

Evaluation is a bucket word. Indeed, its appeal lies partly in its ambiguity.   It embraces commitments to measuring impacts, developing programmes, testing theories, social criticism, and empowerment. In this chapter we will operate with a conventional definition of evaluation implicit in most governmental policy formulations.   Evaluation comprises periodic, independent and 'objective' review of a policy or a programme, and addresses, as a minimum, issues of output, impact, effectiveness, efficiency and relevance (Vanheukelen, 1994).

North America

Programme evaluation was introduced for the first time on a systematic basis in the United States during the 1960s by Robert MacNamara as a budget and management tool. Corporate approaches to planning, programming and budgeting, which reached their zenith in the States and elsewhere during the 1970s, did not survive, but the use of evaluation as a fiscal and management instrument remained.

The Reagan years were marked by a sharp fall in the evaluation capacity of federal programmes. There was a 22 per cent decline in the number of staff in agency programme evaluation units between 1980 and 1984, and an additional cut of 12 per cent between 1984 and 1988. Funding dropped 37 per cent in real terms from 1980 to 1984. There is no indication that investment in programme evaluation showed any meaningful overall increase from 1988 to 1992, when the Clinton administration came to power faced with a serious federal budget deficit and a number of potentially explosive domestic problems which were likely to intensify concern with the effective management of federal programmes (United States General Accounting Office (GAO), 1992).

The United States General Accounting Office called for a rebuild of lost evaluation capacity in 1988 and 1992 (GAO 1988, 1992a, 1992b, 1992c), and registered its disquiet that executive federal agencies varied widely in the extent to which they carried out evaluation. Three problems were identified. The effects of important programmes were often unknown, some agencies were poorly informed about programme implementation, and agencies sometimes relied on flawed studies or ignored sound analyses. In the US health and personal social services fields Medicare costs have spiralled, public confidence in the social security programme is low, and there have been problems over the failure of individual states to implement key reforms such as the 1988 Family Support Act, because of caseload increases and constraints on state budgets. Child welfare programmes also need reform in the face of growing rates of child poverty. One effect of these problems has been to increase pressure for goal-oriented performance standards, and thus has led to a strong managerial influence on all evaluation.

More upbeat noises about evaluation have been made during the mid 1990s. Eleanor Chelimsky, past Assistant Comptroller General of the US General Accounting Office, expressed confidence that,

> Bounding back from reports of an early death in 1980, we find, in 1994, a renascent evaluation profession moving toward expanded use in new topical areas, with broader experience, stronger practice, and...some real legislative support (along with a far-reaching executive initiative called the National Performance Review) behind it
>
> (Chelimsky, 1994: 1).

Chelimsky is also President of the American Evaluation Association, and the 1990s saw the growth of evaluation associations in Central and South America, Canada, Australia, Europe and the United Kingdom. We will discuss the reasons for this renewed optimism in Chapters Five and Nine.

Europe

The way in which the evaluation function is organised in European countries varies, particularly in the extent to which it is decentralised, as in Denmark, or centralised, as in France and increasingly in Britain and Holland. Evaluation is only gradually finding acceptance in southern European countries.

Inspired by US experience, the French government introduced a global evaluation initiative in 1970, which required each ministry to evaluate ministerial policies and actions. This resulted in a period of intense evaluation, and some 500 studies were completed between 1970 and 1982 when the programme was abandoned. A law on the evaluation of public policies, passed in 1990, created an instrument consisting of an inter-ministerial committee, a national fund for the development of evaluation, and a scientific evaluation council (Bletsas, 1994). Those involved in this structure take decisions on which evaluations should be launched, enable financing of agreed evaluations, ensure the quality of evaluations, and follow up their results.

The United Kingdom has the longest experience of evaluation of public policy within the European Community. The Treasury has published guides for managers and for setting targets and measuring performance, but the responsibility for carrying out evaluations lies with the spending departments. The growth of the performance culture and managing by effectiveness models has shaped welfare services evaluation in both the public and independent sectors.

The evaluation of government policies in the Netherlands reflects to some degree the French experience. An inter-ministerial Commission for the Development of Policy Analysis was located in the Ministry of Finance in 1971. This centralised system was abandoned in 1983, and ministers were given responsibility for their own evaluation activities. However, in 1991 a government reform of evaluation activities was introduced, and evaluation co-ordination units were created within ministries, along with a strengthened Division of Policy Analysis. The Luxembourg-based Court of Auditors supervises the implementation of this reform.

Evaluation in the German government is decentralised to the different ministries, and has progressed patchily. The view within the European Commission is that this is due in part to a general mistrust of evaluation that characterises the administrative services, and 'the constant tendency to use evaluation studies for political ends' (Bletsas, 1994: 6).

The European commission

An increase in evaluation resources and interest has been apparent within the European Union during the 1990s. The Financial Regulations were changed in 1990, and now provide for the evaluation of all Union policies. The Maastricht Treaty in the following year included a specific provision that the Commission should strengthen its system for evaluating Community legislation, and the European Parliament in 1993 passed a resolution in which it requested the Commission to demonstrate its commitment to evaluating every policy. An international expert group reported to the Commission in 1995, highlighting the principal weaknesses of the present situation, and suggesting remedies.

There are however limitations to evaluation within the European Union which stem from a variety of causes. The EU has been the subject of allegations of waste and fraud, its organisational culture is resistant to change, and there is widespread concern about the lack of transparency of decisions. Budgets are often protected, which in turn makes evaluation of limited immediate impact. Member states also act in ways which serve to circumscribe the quality of evaluations. For instance, net *contributors* to the community budget tend to favour evaluation of *other* states, and often the dominant position of one partner imposes its own rationality and objectives on others. European evaluation funds are hard to control, once they have arrived with the national or regional authorities to which they have been allocated. Finally, evaluation is unlikely to prove a panacea. Evaluation reports will seldom prove conclusive or undisputed, and wider political objectives will always - and in many cases rightly - prove a telling counter to arguments based on considerations of evaluation and cost effectiveness.

National and regional diversity in evaluation work will continue to influence practice. Within social work, occupational, professional, policy and relevant academic discipline boundaries all vary from one country to another, with the consequence that common ground may be more apparent than real, and definitional disputes over problems such as homelessness clog collaborative evaluation enterprise. These wider considerations provide the backcloth against which we must set the mandates for evaluation in UK welfare services in the following pages.

Evaluation in a performance culture

Fiscal control and programme management are the tightly coupled rationales for government level instruments aimed at policy and programme evaluation. Since the mid 1980s the languages of cost-effectiveness, service-user satisfaction, empowerment, management by effectiveness, quality, service contracts, partnership, staff supervision, financial decentralisation and targeted measurement have permeated the planning, management and delivery of British social services.

The community care changes included requirements for assessment of service quality via Community Care Plans. Plans must include arrangements for quality assurance and systems for safeguarding service standards, including complaints procedures, and must demonstrate user involvement. The Children Act, 1989, led to a plethora of guidance which endeavoured to make social work transactions more visible, and susceptible to monitoring and evaluation against success criteria, and all of these developments have been accompanied by the strengthening of the Social Services Inspectorate.

Government links with agencies and projects in the voluntary sector were subject to Home Office scrutiny in 1990 (Home Office, 1990). The result of this underestimated exercise is that spending departments funding these programmes are expected to obtain explicit evidence from agencies and projects about the outcomes of funding. The Probation Service, through the annually updated Home Office Three Year Plans, has introduced key indicators to measure the performance of probation officers (Home Office, 1994; 1995b).

The Central Council for Education and Training in Social Work requires that social workers in Britain should be able to 'contribute to the maintenance, critical evaluation and development of (their) own professional practice, knowledge and values' (CCETSW, 1995). Whether evaluation is treated as a specific core competence (as in the original requirements for the Diploma in Social Work, CCETSW, 1989), or as a dimension which permeates every competence (as is implied in the current Rules and Requirements), is of secondary importance to the larger picture of increasing expectations that social workers must demonstrate effective practice within organisations. A corresponding sharpening of expectations that social workers should be able to achieve demonstrably effective practice has taken place through the accreditation standards of the Council on Social Work Education in America.

Evaluation: understanding and action

Much of what we have described so far has not been about social work as such, but about larger political and governmental canvases of finance and policy. Evaluation involves both ways of understanding and agendas for action, which are set against this political canvas. How social workers resolve their relative commitments to understanding and action will lend perspective to this wider canvas.

'The intellectual taint of boredom and triviality sticks...to empirical research' (Bulmer, 1982: 30). Martin Bulmer's conclusion doubtless embraces the opinions of many social workers. Yet within applied social research and, by extension, evaluation, fundamental challenges have been made in recent years to earlier ideas about the role of such research and evaluation. There has been a move from the natural sciences towards the view that research and evaluation have more in common with the humanities. This humanist approach has been accompanied by an increasing emphasis on qualitative evaluation, and by a questioning of the traditional boundaries between evaluation and politics. Such politicisation of evaluation has proceeded on the general argument that, because all evaluation is inevitably fashioned by ideology, values and epistemology, then ideological commitment should be openly adopted.

As a preamble to mapping attempts to integrate understanding and action, it may help to broadly distinguish different kinds of evaluation in social work. At the risk of oversimplifying, we can crudely differentiate the *methodology* and the *purpose* of social work evaluation (cf Howe, 1988). Methodology, in the sense of a general strategy for knowing about social work, may be either *humanist* or *empiricist*. Humanist evaluation is likely to adopt qualitative methods of inquiry and to stress the importance of discovering the meaning of events to the participants. Hence 'process' and the way in which meanings are constructed through negotiation are liable to figure largely. Within this approach we will find strong relativists but also those who believe evaluation uncovers real knowledge about the world. Empiricism is 'a conception of social research involving the production of accurate data - meticulous, precise, generalisable - in which the data themselves constitute an end of the research' (Bulmer, 1982: 31). The emphasis is more likely to be on outcomes, as well as on sharp descriptive accounts of processes. Quantitative methods will figure more centrally. Inquiry will be seen as primarily factual and the task of such evaluation regarded as the production of facts for use.

The word 'purpose' is perhaps too pretentious for what I intend as the second dimension of social work evaluation. Evaluation may address issues of either *practice* or *service*. *Service evaluation* focuses on understanding and/or changing ways in which services are fashioned and delivered within organisations. *Practice evaluation* investigates direct, face-to-face practice, which may be understood separately from its agency context, for example as a method of intervention.

Two caveats are in order. *First*, this is a typology, and we should not expect to discover that all or even most evaluations fall neatly into one or other category. In practice, better evaluations will often include elements of service evaluation and practice evaluation. And because humanist or empiricist evaluations comprise elements that cluster together for pragmatic reasons as well as those derived from social science, many evaluations will fall somewhere in the middle of this continuum. The examples suggested below could, for these reasons, very well be placed elsewhere. *Second*, the terms 'service', 'practice', 'humanist' and 'empiricist' are not introduced as either 'hurrah' or 'boo' words. To illustrate, we will see in Chapter Six that the tendency of social workers and those who write about social work to use 'positivism' and associated words like 'empiricist' as 'boo' words has diluted the possibility for critical assessment. Although we will subsequently criticise heavily some aspects of empiricist service evaluation (Chapter Five) and practice evaluation (Chapter Nine), there is no inherent reason why they should be declared in advance as out of court and *non grata*.

Figure 2.1 demonstrates the four types of evaluation that ensue when we distinguish between the methodology and purpose of evaluation.

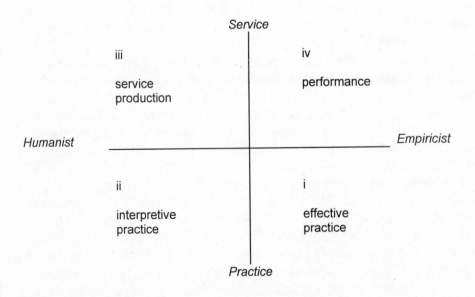

Figure 2.1   Social work evaluations

Examples of evaluation as *effective practice* include practice which draws on research about task-centred work, crisis intervention, and single system evaluations utilising approximations to experiments (eg Bloom, 1993). Evaluations based on critical theory and feminist methodology will fall within *interpretive practice*, as will some evaluation of groupwork or community groups and practice influenced by studies of client and carer perspectives on social work. More recent studies of user involvement in social service planning and implementation (eg Barnes and Wistow, 1992) belong more properly in the *service production* 'corner' of evaluation, along with evaluations of the street level implementation of policy by social workers, and studies of organisational process (eg Pithouse, 1987). Larger scale programme evaluations, much of the research carried out at research units such as the Personal Social Services Research Unit at Kent University on the production of welfare, and the majority of quality assurance research can be described as *performance evaluation*.

Evaluating in practice may fall almost anywhere in this schematic view of evaluation. It obviously may be oriented towards effective practice or interpretive practice, and Participatory Action Research, which we outline below, can best be understood as a variety of service production evaluation. Practice monitoring and some 'gatekeeping' evaluation, of the kind described later in this book, include elements of performance evaluation.

Recent debate about the relationship between understanding and action has been fuelled but not invented by developments in the social sciences that draw inspiration from a humanist perspective, and which are committed to qualitative methods of inquiry (Denzin and Lincoln, 1994; Hammersley, 1995). Once translated to social work practice, the position taken by social workers on this issue will prove probably the most influential ground rule constraining the way in which they view the character of evaluating in practice (Sheldon, 1987). There are five main options currently on offer for squaring the circle of understanding and action. They are, evaluation as applied research, evaluation as action research, practitioner research, participatory inquiry, and advocacy evaluation. Clear distinctions do not exist between these approaches, and the boundaries are frequently fuzzy. Action research and advocacy evaluation each have two distinct strands. Action research 'as a way of generating knowledge about a social system while, at the same time, trying to change it' (Elden and Chisholm, 1993: 121), is associated in Britain especially with the Tavistock Institute.   In the late 1960's action research came to have a quite separate association through the work of the American Poverty Programme, and the introduction of programmes of positive discrimination in education and through the Home Office funded Community Development Projects (Specht, 1976).   Advocacy evaluation includes critical evaluation based on feminist methodology and other directly anti-discriminatory methodologies, but also includes participatory research stemming from the evaluation of Third World development programmes.   Brief outlines of each of these solutions to the problem of understanding and action are pencilled in, in the following paragraphs.   Their contribution to evaluating in practice is assessed in Chapter Six.

Applied research

Thoroughgoing empiricism in the social sciences has often been characterised by an optimism about the potential of applying facts to social ills.   There is a direct line in British social administration from Charles Booth via Richard Titmuss to Peter Townsend, and political commitment and scholarly research have effectively coexisted within the Fabian tradition of empiricism.   Pressure group rhetoric and research also falls within an empiricist tradition.

Bulmer (1982) suggests that in addition to the empiricist model we must also distinguish the 'engineering' and the 'enlightenment' models.   The engineering model assumes a problem defined by policy makers, resulting in a product which is for policy and not for social science. Large scale programme evaluation and small, one-off commissioned or in-house evaluations are contrasting examples of engineering research.   The advocates of the enlightenment model take a longer term and perhaps less optimistic view about the practical impacts of research; and they argue that research is unlikely to have a *direct* impact on policy or practice, but that it will provide an *orienting* function which, over a longer period, will influence the way decision makers define social problems. Bulmer suggests that race relations research functioned in this way, by providing a new angle of vision on a problem.

Evaluation defined in this way as applied research contains a cluster of associated arguments about what *kind* of research is needed, how it should be *organised*, and how it should be *utilised*. There have been several efforts to identify what kind of research is needed if it is to be readily applied.   For example, Seidl (1980) suggested that for a research problem to be relevant to social work practice it should meet the following requirements:

- variables which can be subject to planned change, rather than non-manipulable variables which the practitioner can do little or nothing about.
- the need of practitioners is for knowledge that can be discovered through research, while recognising that not all knowledge can be discovered in this way.
- problem intelligibility, ie a research problem that is cast in the language of the utiliser.
- timeliness. 'There are many situations in which quick and dirty is better than long and clean' (Seidl, 1980: 56).
- space specificity. If it is to be useful, research cannot afford to ignore local variability and context, simply because it has little theoretical relevance.

There is a continuing interest in research for application in social work through a revival of tough-minded empiricism which claims that the pessimistic conclusion that 'nothing works' which was drawn from the evaluation research in the 1960s and 1970s was derived from a mixture of inadequate research and faulty argument. Practitioners and social work academics committed to the integration of practice and research to form empirically based practice, generally believe that 'the key to integration lies in the conception of the measurement process' (Blythe and Tripodi, 1989: 14). In other words, the solution to the problem of social work effectiveness is seen as primarily a technical one. The evidence so far is that this promotion of empirical practice has yet to bring social workers and researchers any closer together.

The distinction between pure and applied research had its most influential statement in the Rothschild report (1971), which continues to shape the way applied research is organised. Applied research is funded through customer/contractor relationships, and it represents the claim by the paying customer for a say in setting the evaluation agenda and some degree of control over what happens to the results.

Concerns that the application of the final research product might prove inadequate have led to a series of government sponsored social work research utilisation and dissemination exercises, and major research charities such as the Rowntree Trust and the Kings Fund place the dissemination and utilisation of findings near the forefront of research sponsorship decisions. A different approach to strengthening research utilisation by practitioners is represented by the efforts of professionals and academics to promote the acquisition of research appraisal skills by social workers (Mencher, 1959; Black, 1993).

The main problem with evaluation viewed as applied research, in particular the empiricist and engineering varieties, is that it is often premised on an assumption that the facts speak for themselves. This over estimates the impact of information on policy and practice, and gives too little weight to the influence of values and ideas (Rein and White, 1981). Evaluating needs a good idea. A social worker is someone with a problem to solve if he/she is anybody.

Action research

Early action research focused on intra-organisational and work life problems.

> Action research aims to contribute both to the practical concerns of people in an immediate problematic situation and to the goals of social science by joint collaboration within a mutually acceptable ethical framework
> (Rapaport, quoted in Elden and Chisholm, 1993: 124).

Action research links solving practical problems with scientific enterprise, thus rejecting the idea of a value-free science. It is carried out in collaboration with those who experience the problem or their representatives, and in this respect recent action research has shifted in the direction of participatory inquiry, where participants are regarded as co-researchers and 'normal science' methods are modified through an increasing stress on 'local knowledge' (Whyte, 1991). There is also a strong commitment to a cyclical process in which evaluation leads to new diagnoses, and to sustainability so that learning continues after the researcher leaves the system. But no one working in the action research tradition would advocate participation as a requirement of all research, and they reject 'participatory dogmatism.' Participation is viewed as essentially an emergent quality of research. 'No-one may mandate in advance that a particular research process will become a fully developed participatory action research project.' Such a view is dismissed as 'both naive and morally suspect' (Greenwood, Whyte and Harkavy, 1993: 176). But on precisely the same grounds 'we also do not think that any action researcher is ever free of the obligation to do whatever is possible to enhance participation' (p180).

A strong organisation focus still characterises action research, although it also has been applied to community groups. This means that the method is very Western oriented; and even when strong participatory ideas emerge, they rarely connect with the interesting work on participatory research presently taking place in Non-Governmental Organisations. Action research has not received much careful consideration within British social work, although its influence is evident in the occasional promotion of self-evaluation in voluntary organisations (Meadows and Turkie, 1988; Robb and Hasen, 1991).

Action research assumed a new identity in the wake of Lyndon Johnson's Poverty Programme. 'The hope of administrators and the despair of academics' (Ruddock, 1981: 66), the core of action research was a statement about the relation between the action and the evaluation. It included an argument to bring the evaluation task into the project at an early stage, so that it did not become a semi-detached add-on. It was also an argument for researchers to be part of the action team. Evaluation was not regarded as being concerned with discipline development but was to be directly responsive to the needs and agenda set by the action programme. Most significantly it represented in many though not all instances (Specht, 1976) an instrumental, activist view of research, where research is viewed as intrinsically a political enterprise. The conventional idea was rejected - of research as at least partly autonomous from practical and political activities. It shared with later advocacy evaluation a commitment to understanding the world by changing it, although it did not typically involve action beneficiaries in the evaluation. Action research had its main impact on social work through the Community Development Projects which were the main vehicle for the radicalisation of community work during the 1970s, and exercised an influence on social work far beyond their scale and five-year time spans.

Practitioner research

Practitioner research shares with action research a determination to change the traditional relationship between programme providers and the evaluation task. However, whereas action research focuses on the relation between evaluators and practitioners, practitioner research has at its core the linked assumptions that practitioners can and should do the evaluation themselves. As McIvor aptly puts it, the starting point...is the twofold belief that practitioners should be encouraged to engage in the evaluation of their own practice and that they possess many of the skills which are necessary to undertake the evaluative task

(McIvor, 1995: 210).

The basic idea that professionals should carry out small-scale research within and on their practice has, of course, a long pedigree, and in professions such as medicine researcher-clinicians have for a long time played a central role in the critical development of knowledge and practice. Social workers whose practice involves co-working with clinicians in medicine and psychiatry have a tradition of practitioner research involvement which is stronger than among those working in mainstream social work. However, there has been a flurry of recent interest in promoting a research-minded, empirical practice (Broad and Fletcher, 1993; Fuller and Petch, 1995). An important difference between practitioner research and mainstream research is that research and practice are usually seen as part of a single whole in practitioner research. At the very minimum, practitioner researchers practise with a spirit of inquiry, seeking to gain increased knowledge and understanding through their practice. Stronger versions of practitioner research include planning and undertaking a small piece of research relevant to practice, or even approaching all social work practice as if it is similar to research in its skills and strategies.

It is not always easy to be precise about the identifying features of practitioner research, and this is partly because it is sometimes defined so broadly that it includes any research so long as it is done by a practitioner (e.g. Broad and Fletcher, 1993). The core of the argument for practitioner research is that research aims and skills have strong points of contact and comparability with social work aims and skills. Feminist writers have argued that 'Research, practice and social action are one unified effort' in which 'the empowerment of oppressed groups and practitioner-researchers occurs simultan-eously' (Swigonski, 1993: 182). Other writers have emphasised that social workers and researchers both use skills such as problem solving, negotiation, effective interviewing and planning, which provide the basis for engaging in research and practice simultaneously as a set of integrated activities, thus making possible an empirically based model of practice. Because of these important points of contact, 'beneficial changes may occur through the results generated by the research but also through participating in the research process itself' (Whittaker and Archer, 1990-1991: 12).

Single system research represents a more clearly defined variety of practitioner research. It is the main operational plank in the empirical practice movement, and proceeds by applying the logic of large-scale group experiments to single cases. Behavioural psychology has provided the main underpinnings of single system research, although its advocates are convinced that the potential and value of the method should not be limited to any one school or theory. The reasons for the steady growth of interest in single system research can be traced to the 1970s and the focus at that time on issues of practice effectiveness which roused heated debates among social workers. The apparently pessimistic implications of experimental studies of social work (eg Meyer, Borgatta and Jones, 1965; Goldberg, 1970; Fischer, 1976) helped to fuel a philosophical attack on logical positivism, but also roused an interest among some practitioners in evaluating their own practice.

> The consequence of this was a body of angry practitioners who were sweating their guts out trying to help people on a day to day basis, and the development of a tradition among some researchers who said that social work practitioners do not know what they are doing, that they should engage in 'empirically based practice
>
> (Austin, 1992: 317).

The use of single system research is likely to grow in Britain, perhaps especially in the field of social work practice with offenders, but misgivings about its behavioural base will continue to limit the spread of an empirically based practice model. Qualitative versions of practitioner self-evaluation are almost entirely non-existent in social work, although Searight's thorough programme of self-evaluative work, which we discuss in Chapter Seven, and Martin's application of oral history methods to social work intervention (Martin, 1995), have gone some way to demonstrating the potential of such a method (Searight, 1988).

Participatory inquiry

We have already seen that the older tradition of action research associated with Lewin has gained new stimulus from a growing interest in participatory methods of inquiry - research *with* people rather than research *on* or *about* people. Claims to be 'participatory' are made by a wide variety of research and evaluation methods, but they can be broadly distinguished according to whether personal or political *change* are seen as the main and perhaps only measure of validity, or whether the development of *understanding* and *knowledge* is also regarded as part of the purpose of the research or evaluation. Evaluation which falls into the first general category is better described as advocacy evaluation, which we discuss below.

One of the clearest cases for participative inquiry has been made by Peter Reason (Reason and Rowan, 1981; Reason, 1988; 1994a; 1994b). He rejects positivist and modernist worldviews on the grounds that they separate the knower and the known. Proceeding on the basis that 'a participative methodology needs to rest on a participative world-view', he is 'much persuaded' that 'the purpose of human inquiry is not so much the search for truth but to *heal*...the alienation...that characterises modern experience' (Reason, 1994a: 1, 10). His methodological solution stems from his belief that 'we can only truly do research *with* persons if we engage with them *as* persons, as co-subjects and thus as co-researchers' (p10).

This approach is quite different from the demythologising approach of deconstruction, which he forcibly criticises as both alienating and relativistic.

> the fashion of deconstructive post-modernism is nihilistic, indeed, is an extension of the alienation of modernism. If voices are just voices and have no claim to truth, the search for voice becomes the search for any old voice; it no longer matters what we say about ourselves (p14).

There are various strands of participatory inquiry, which go under names like Co-operative Inquiry, Action Science, Action Inquiry, and Participatory Action Research and are associated with the writings of Heron, Whyte, Schon, Argyris and Tarbert. At the risk of over-simplifying, the main recurring themes are:

- subjectivity. 'Valid human inquiry essentially requires full partic-ipation in the creation of personal and social knowings' (Reason, 1994b: 332).
- the models of 'normal science' are, to varying degrees, supplanted by an emphasis on the value of lay knowledge, and by the use of less conventional forms of methods.
- knowledge arises *out of* action and is *for* action. The interest does not lie in developing an applied science but in a genuine science of action.
- knowledge is tested in live-action contexts.

- unlike more explicit advocacy evaluation approaches, the egalitarianism of these methods is tempered with a reliance on leadership.

A number of imaginative examples of participatory inquiry have been carried out, and because the potential of applying these methods to social work is considerable, there will be a continuing expansion of interest in this field in the next few years. Expectations of user involvement in the community care field also guarantee a stage on which participatory inquiry can play a significant role.

Advocacy evaluation

Participatory inquiry tails back to older action research traditions and forward to full blown advocacy evaluation - a term which links together anti-discriminatory evaluation promoted most vocally through feminist methodology, and participatory research originating in recent practice in Third World development research.

Feminist work on research methodology has radical implications for evaluating in practice. The literature is extensive, increasingly diverse and rapidly developing. Useful accounts mapping feminism in its relation to qualitative research have been given by Warren (1988), Reinharz (1992) and Olesen (1994), but with the reservation that 'qualitative feminist research is not homogenous but highly differentiated' (Olesen, 1994: 168). Feminist positions start from the proposition that when evaluating practice the practitioner must ask questions which make sense within women's experience, and must evaluate practice *for* women. Some feminist researchers believe that this principle requires a strong participative commitment, and have worked with people as co-researcher participants in the interests of empowering rather than exploiting them. Research is seen as being '*for* the subjects of research, to advance their causes' and therefore researchers need to 'work towards the active participation of members of oppressed groups in every phase of their research activities' (Swigonski, 1993: 178). Social workers engaged in anti-discriminatory evaluation are invited to demonstrate a 'conscious partiality with those who are marginalised or invisible, or whose experiences have been distorted by traditional research', which exhibits a 'conceptual imperialism' based on male power, and is 'white, eurocentric, heterosexual and able-bodied' (Humphries and Truman, 1994: 1,3). Anti-discriminatory evaluation requires 'an active involvement in challenging assumptions based on unequal social relations, through reflexive, explicitly committed participation in the process of social change' (p14).

Perhaps the most important challenge raised by this argument is that it changes the *process* of evaluation and not simply the *outcome*. In this respect it has much in common with participatory research, a variety of advocacy evaluation which owes its main origin to efforts to bring Third World development *practice* closer to development *research* (Chambers, 1983; Marsden and Oakley, 1990; Pratt and Boyden 1985; Edwards, 1989; Booth, 1994). There has been a shift in social development evaluation towards a qualitative approach, caused by changing understandings of the meaning of social development which emphasise grassroots involvement (Marsden and Oakley, 1990). Michael Edwards, who has worked within Non-Governmental Organisations (NGO's)'s, presents the argument persuasively. He complains about the absence of strong links between understanding and action, and lists the problems as follows:

> the 'professionalisation' of development studies and the devaluation of popular knowledge; the values and attitudes of researchers and practitioners that prevent them from working as equals; the control of knowledge by elites; and a failure to unite understanding, action, relevance and participation
>
> (Edwards, 1989: 133).

He complains that the thousands of experts and ex-patriates, together with Third World elites which 'mimic the behaviour of their counterparts in Europe and North America' (p119), create and perpetuate a series of divorces, the most complete of which 'lies between research output and the subjects of this research - poor people themselves. The barriers created by jargon, language, literacy, price, availability and method create a situation where people are denied access to the information which is supposed to concern them.' While he is insistent that method has not been the only problem, he nonetheless insists that 'participatory research is the vehicle for understanding and changing the world simultaneously' (128). In the telling words of a Mexican proverb which he quotes, 'we make the path by walking it.'

There has been some heat generated at western colonising of this explicitly liberationist strategy (Cervinskas, 1991). However, it raises a series of inescapable questions which transfer with equal potency to evaluations by social workers. First, what do we mean by claiming that evaluation is 'relevant'? The meaning of relevance is one of the most controversial debates in social development research (Booth, 1994). Second, is *relevant* evaluation the same as *participatory* evaluation? Third, what is the relationship between grassroots evaluating and 'higher level' evaluation? One of the dangers of recent post-Marxist shifts to enthusiastic adoption of explanations based on culture, diversity, agency and actor constructions is that the relationship between the micro level of individual practice and the structural level is ignored. How can social workers be committed to evaluation at the micro level and still keep the macro issues firmly on the table? The questions raised by people such as Chambers and Edwards - 'unashamedly polemical born out of years of frustration' (Edwards, 1994: 279) - are in some ways more sharply uncomfortable for social workers than the more global statements that characterise feminist methodology. They are certainly more neglected by social workers.

Evaluating in practice: understanding and action

We began this passage by emphasising that clear distinctions between these various efforts to integrate understanding and action are not possible. There are important internal differences that make thumb nail sketches of participatory inquiry and advocacy evaluation especially hazardous. This is partly because writers are engaged in conscious, political claims-making, and partly because there are several key dimensions that cut across different approaches. For example, the issue of normal science versus what is sometimes called new paradigm science cuts across almost all these areas of evaluation. Second, the widely different ideas about what counts as 'relevance' also risk jeopardising efforts at summary statements about the relation of knowledge and practice. This has been most clearly debated in the area of advocacy evaluation, and we return to the theme in Chapter Six. Third, there is an easy confusion of language. For example, *action*-oriented *evaluation* is a very different kettle of fish from *actor*-oriented *research*. Fourth, the nature and impact of any particular action-oriented evaluation is difficult to identify because evaluation may have indirect effects, or may have unknown or unknowable effects. The debate in participatory research about 'scaling up' and the relation between micro research and macro level research is a good example of this problem. However, having sounded these cautions, it is possible to suggest a rough sorting (Figure 2.2) based on the immediate *purpose* of the evaluation, the immediate *target*, and with whom the immediate *responsibility* for evaluation lies.

	Applied Research	Action Research (Lewin)	Action Research (poverty)	Practitioner Research	Participatory Inquiry	Advocacy Evaluation (A/D)	Advocacy Evaluation (PR)
A) Purpose							
Understanding	(✓)			(✓)			
Action via understanding	✓	✓	✓	✓	✓	(✓)	✓
Direct action			✓	(✓)		✓	✓
B) Responsibility							
Practitioner				✓		✓	✓
Expert researcher	✓	✓	✓		✓		
Shared		(✓)	✓	(✓)	✓	✓	✓
C) Target							
Service development and planning	✓	✓	✓	(✓)		✓	(✓)
Service implementation and outcomes	✓	✓	✓	✓	✓	(✓)	
Direct personal practice				(✓)	(✓)	✓	✓

✓   =   primary
(✓)   =   secondary

Figure 2.2   Evaluation and action

We will describe fully in Chapter Six what evaluating in practice entails. However, compared with the strategies in Figure 2.2, the *purpose* of evaluating in practice is action through understanding, for which the practitioner takes the primary *responsibility*, and evaluation is *targeted* at direct personal practice. Our earlier caveats about classifications of evaluating strategies apply equally here. In particular, evaluating in practice cannot be seen as a single fixed entity, but issues of 'scaling up' and relevance need careful work, along with the emergent participatory dimension which must be part of all practice evaluation.

In this chapter we have explored the governmental politics, welfare policies, and strategies of understanding and action which provide the context and scene in which social workers carry out their practice. We hold these in one hand for the next three chapters while we shift ground to explore what social workers believe and say about their present practice. How do social workers decide whether they are practising well or not? What evidence do they draw on in reaching those decisions? How do their evaluations relate to those of service users, carers, colleagues, and other practitioners?

3   Practitioners talk

Thou shalt not sit
With statisticians nor commit
A social science.

W H Auden *('Under Which Lyre')*

Don't ask me to evaluate people - that just clutters my mind.

Social worker

You evaluate because you have to. It's not something that excites you in your work at all. If something is going well you enjoy evaluating and looking back, 'Yeah, that had been great'. If it's not going well it's a burden because showing anything and evaluation - it's not very constructive.

Probation officer

Evaluating in practice must be relevant. If it is not to be regarded by practitioners as an appendix to the real business of social work practice, then it must make sense within the contexts of existing practice. How do social workers know if they are doing well or not in their day-to-day practice? In what ways do social workers carry out evaluation as part of their day-to-day practice? The problem, of course, is that we have only the slightest knowledge of if and how social workers evaluate their practice. Both senses of the chapter title - the *substance* of what practitioners have to say about their evaluating practices, and the *ways* in which they talk, the attitudes and beliefs they reveal - provide the starting point for the themes of this book. If the suggestions on evaluating in practice, put forward later in the book, are themselves to be evaluable, then we need to do something to fill in this empirical void. It is for these reasons that we step aside in this chapter and listen to the accounts that practitioners give of their evaluating practices. They should be read in that light. They provide, as we have said already, part of the missing but essential empirical connections for developing an evaluating in practice that is not decontextualised or imposed from the outside. The evidence is drawn from lengthy tape recorded interviews with fifteen recently qualified social work students, practice teachers, and experienced practitioners, practising in a range of social work agencies in England and Wales, and working with individuals and families, groups and community groups.

Customary approaches to the question of whether and how social workers evaluate their practice have until very recently been very different from the one adopted here. Whether social workers evaluate their practice has been assumed to require, especially in much American social work, answers to questions such as: Do they carry out discrete, empirical evaluations within their practice? Do they utilise single case/single system evaluation designs to understand likely cause and effect relations in their work? Have they applied training in evaluation methods acquired in schools of social work? Are the components of practice operationalised so that their work can subsequently be described and assessed in measurable terms? Do they routinely use measurement instruments to test the efficacy of their practice inputs?

There are obvious strengths to this approach. It demands a mental rigour, precision and concern for testability which are sometimes lacking in social work practice, and also presses social workers to think through the relationship between evaluating and intervention in a way that is still strange to most social workers. We return to the possible uses of single case evaluation in Chapter Nine, but we can say now that the upshot and essence of this debate is fairly unanimous. Pleas for an empirical practice fall short because most social workers do not make extensive use of systematic evaluation methods, even when they have been trained in their application on qualifying courses. Furthermore, agency managements provide scant encouragement for such evaluation, either in resources or through supervision.

A different approach is called for if we are to provide an information base to foster ways of evaluating practice that make sense to the practitioner. Penka and Kirk (1991) concluded from a study of New York social workers that social workers *do* evaluate their practices, but that a gap between practitioners and researchers may stem in part from different mindsets. In the minds of practitioners there appeared to be a sharp distinction between formal single subject design studies and the general evaluative tasks in which they routinely engage. An alternative research form is needed, 'one that is exploratory rather than confirmatory, building models of evaluation from the practitioner's own accounts rather than superimposing an ideal model and testing for conformity' (Elks and Kirkhart, 1993: 555).

The core of these pages is the stories told by practitioners, in which they were asked to reflect on their knowing-in-practice, their tacit knowledge, and to review their understanding of what was happening. Talking about and doing evaluation are, while distinct, interactive. What follows is thus not simply a retelling of data. Telling and living aspects of our lives inevitably interlock.

Evaluation with a capital 'E'

Almost every social worker we spoke to distinguished two subjectively real kinds of evaluation. These were 'evaluation proper' and self-evaluation of work with service users for whom they were responsible.

> I tend to think of evaluation *proper*, in inverted commas, as being more to do with facts and figures.

> I actually in-built my own kind of evaluation. I'd use a kind of informal system of measurement to see whether I'm doing what *I* see as being a *good job*. And that's not necessarily what the agency would say, 'You're doing a good job'.

1	part of a widespread change of culture in social work which emphasises performance
2	experienced as a scrutiny from above
3	formal, planned and takes place occasionally rather than all the time
4	relatively time consuming
5	measured quantitatively and not qualitatively
6	responds to expectations created from above and outside direct practice
7	focuses on an agenda of service level concerns rather than direct practice concerns

Figure 3.1   The identifying characteristics of 'evaluation proper'

Each kind of evaluation has its own characteristic hallmarks, which, apart from one or two important cross-over points, represent entirely distinctive sets of commitments, activities and attitudes. The distinctives of 'Evaluation proper' are summarised in Figure 3.1.

In Chapter Five we will consider 'Evaluation with a Capital E' and the influence of agency settings on practice evaluations, and pick up practitioners' stories from this point.

Self-evaluating in action

There was a widely held consensus on the following features of evaluation in action (Figure 3.2).

1	Quality and worth, and not quantity
2	Personal immediacy, informal, private and subjective. Sometimes described as 'on your feet' evaluation
3	Not part of the core of social work practice skills, but is a marginal 'add-on' to practice. The language of evaluation is 'foreign' to practice
4	Requires long-term perspective for results to be seen
5	Assumes a social work practice in which evaluation has to draw on complex evidence that is not easy to interpret
6	Assumes a social work practice in which progress is typically achieved by slow, incremental steps
7	Connects with core personal commitments and values
8	Sometimes draws on the framework of 'evaluation proper' to provide a 'scaffolding' for personal evaluation

Figure 3.2   Identifying characteristics of self-evaluation

Evaluating rarely comes up explicitly in conversation within agencies, and there was no ready made practice vocabulary into which it fitted. It was something that 'you just don't think about on a daily basis' and is 'not the word that would be bandied about the office with my colleagues'.

Social workers repeatedly said that 'It's not a word that we use'. If they did discuss it, then it was something done implicitly, through coffee break conversations about whether someone had done the right thing in a particular situation. When talking about evaluating they resorted to various linguistic approximations. Appraisal, assessment, planning, review, supervision, reflection, gatekeeping, judgement, thinking time and, occasionally, research were the 'in-a-way' approximations that social workers resorted to as a way of giving accounts of what evaluation meant for them.

Because evaluation was not part of social workers' mental picture of practice skills, it became a marginal 'add-on' which fitted uncomfortably with normal practice, as 'a separate skill':

> It's something that you've always added on to your work...It's not, sort of a natural part of your work.... you realise it's not used that much, and it's very much something added on...it's just tagged on at the end.

This had several consequences. First it readily gets put to the bottom of the pile. Second, evaluation becomes seen as a special interest rather than a core practice. 'It's something that basically you have to want to do yourself. In terms of doing your own evaluation that is something that is purely down to the individual'. Third, if it is not an individual's special interest, it is likely to be seen as something that has to be done as a chore, as illustrated in the quotation from the probation officer at the head of the chapter. A common, although not universal, response by social workers was to assume that, because of pressure of work, 'crisis work' could not be evaluated. It followed that 'You don't really think about evaluation on a day-to-day basis unless it's a long-term case'.

This long-term view was important. It provided a perspective from which to hold on to a sense of purpose and direction. It enabled social workers to avoid getting snared in insoluble problems, and gave a balanced view of the positives.

Evaluation was made more difficult in the eyes of these social workers because of what they assumed and believed to be the *nature of practice* and the possibility of *progress*. Social work practice was viewed as essentially complex and elusive, with progress being achieved through small, incremental steps with occasional unpredictable jumps. Evaluation, to make sense, had to accommodate itself to this reality. 'You've got different conflicting philosophies around... it's just a very messy complicated business.' The underlying reason for this complexity lies partly in the nature of the evidence. A probation officer concluded that evaluation is 'difficult because it's very complex, and because the things you are measuring sometimes aren't tangible.'

Practice not only involves making sense of complex evidence, but is viewed by most social workers as a slow, at times painfully so, incremental process. 'Coming to a compromise, that's what it's all about', as one social worker put it, describing a case that had gone well. Official Home Office Probation targets may seem demanding but practitioners are more likely to view their work as 'bit by bit, the behaviourist thing', and 'not to change everything so that they never offend again, that's usually not too realistic.' Slow *practice* progress was echoed in step-by-step *evaluation*. Evaluation, is 'a continuous slow process, a slow accumulation of knowledge...it's almost in parallel with the work itself.'

Evaluation might appear from these accounts to be a largely piecemeal, private, opportunist and marginal activity, limited by the realities of practice and without a coherent framework. This would be to overlook that, while evaluating in day-to-day action is seen as a marginal *skill*, it connects with deeply held personal commitments and *values*, associated with a 'general *predisposition* to have your work looked at critically.' A striking instance of the relevance of basic, personal values was evident in the account of a black social worker, describing her work with a woman service user.

> I feel very committed to my job because it's part of me, it's part of the struggle working with women, women's issues, talking about our oppression, talking about our coming into a strange country, finding it difficult to get a job... All that for me is part of my life, not just my job.

> If (employer) comes and tells you, 'You have to tell me what you are doing', you have to say 'Well, I came into work today, I took time off in lieu and I...', you know what I mean. And then you think they don't take into account all the work I'm doing when it's not written down on paper. But I do understand and I know that I have to evaluate my work. It's really difficult when it's something which you feel very committed to. You think, 'What do they know about me and my commitment?' It's something you can't write down on paper, and something you can't ever rate'.

Social workers sometimes illustrated how a more personal self-evaluation approach provided a sense of perspective at difficult moments. 'For me my evaluating skills are caught up with what I believe, and the reasons I believe I'm doing this...I want to *protect* and help *children,* and *families*, and I want them to get a good service.' For example, when a client invokes complaints procedures,

'I suppose that does make us evaluate our work, and it makes us think, "Well, yeah, could I have done that differently, is that OK?".'

Preoccupations about evaluation can on occasion lead to deeply pessimistic conclusions. Talking about mental health practice, one social worker reflected,

> We have to tolerate seeing them suffering, and it's quite hard sometimes. It takes a lot out of you emotionally to deal with this client group because you get the odd success but you get so much in the way of failure within the system. It's a bit like a drop in the ocean...You feel the pain that these people go through, and it really does touch raw nerves within you, it's a very painful bit of social work, mental health...it's just so difficult. We're in a twilight world where we're just sort of ferreting around.

We have only seen a very small part of the picture so far - the straight edges and corners of the jigsaw - but already we can draw some tentative conclusions. There is a generally negative perception of agency led evaluations coupled to a widely held acceptance - if on occasion with grim resignation - that a culture of evaluation is here to stay for the foreseeable future.

But most social workers feel patently ill-equipped to develop an evaluative stance that they can accept with integrity as part of their practice. 'We're dreadful at actually evaluating our own work, dreadful,' was a comment that could be multiplied many times over.

A very different account was presented by one respondent, whose approach was to combat the political *abuses* of evaluation strategies rather than their political *nature*. While he criticised the emphasis on quantitative outcomes as a 'fetish', and talked about ways in which performance rates never carry a straightforward interpretation, he concluded that 'evaluation of practice is such a good tool, such a good thing to develop, to be conscious of, that it outweighs the sub-agendas that exist.'

But this view of evaluating was exceptional. The normal picture, as we have seen, was that evaluating in practice is at present marginal and marginalised. 'It's not something that excites you', with the consequence that the commitment, even of enthusiasts, easily withers. Good practice is thus always at risk.

> It's not seen as a priority. Your priority is to do your PSR and get it to the court, out of the way. Evaluating is 'Oh yeah, I'd better do it just in case'. But if it's given priority from the top down, then I think more would be done with it.

We can draw two conclusions from practitioners' accounts thus far. First, social workers *do* evaluate. Second, while evaluating is pervasive it is also troublesome, almost chronically so. As we subsequently map evaluating in practice competencies, we will find occasion to make repeated connections between how evaluating *is* done and how it *may* be done. The traffic between them will not be one way. Actual practice will many times provide a stimulus and correction to practice prescription.

Strategies for good and bad practice

How do practitioners account for practice which goes well and that which goes badly? How do they *know* whether their work is going well or not? Social workers were asked to identify examples of their work, which had gone well and which had not gone well, and to reflect on how such judgements were reached. Two general questions were considered. First, what evaluation *strategy* do social workers employ? What basic essentials need to be in place if work is to have a chance of going well? Second, what *evidence* counts in deciding how well a piece of work has gone? Social workers displayed an unexpected consensus on evaluation strategies, which were made up of the elements in Figure 3.3.

1	An implicit 'game plan'. This comprises
	• the ability to exercise a controlling influence over clients and other key actors
	• a purposeful and 'constructive' practice strategy
	• keeping practice in the rules of the 'ball game'
2	'Knowing' the target of their interventions. This special knowledge consists of
	• constant watchfulness
	• knowledge built on life experience and professional experience
	• a sense of 'timing'
3	'Rules' for recognising a good client
4	Recognising the significant parts played by
	• unpredictable 'luck'
	• factors that mitigate against blame for poor practice

Figure 3.3   Strategies for evaluating used by practitioners

A game plan

The possession of a game plan depends, using the terms of our respondents, on three issues - keeping or losing control of the work, carrying out 'constructive' practice, and 'staying in the ball park'. 'I don't, like, come into work and think, "Right, today I'm going to evaluate that situation"...I have a kind of game plan in my head which I just *do'*. This social worker went on to explain,

> This probably sounds a bit naive to you, but I think most social workers, or *good* social workers rather, know their capabilities, know their skills, know what they should be doing and they get on with it.

Having a game plan makes control and composure possible - a 'sort of juggling act'. A social worker listed the juggled items in a case that had gone well.

> I felt I successfully worked with the mum, both the dads...the mother's father...enabling the mum...working very closely with the foster carers...with the nursery...with the family unit...working with the adoptive family, encouraging and enabling them...

On the contrary, when work goes badly, social workers repeatedly described it as a loss of, or a failure to gain, control. A social worker who found himself 'in a heavy flow tide...being dragged along with it, having no control over what's actually happening' described a case conference in which

> It became quite out of hand, quite hostile and aggressive. I was trying to chair the meeting as well as play an active part. I was trying to keep the focus firmly on the welfare of the child. I don't think I was able to do that as well as I would have liked.

This control, or appropriate influence, as one social worker explained it, was frequently described in terms of the second dimension of a 'game plan', being *'constructive'* in practice. The question of constructiveness most often emerged when social workers were giving accounts of work that had gone badly. The absence of clear assessments, plans and objectives was a frequent self-criticism. Poor assessment and planning leads in turn to aimless intervention.

> I never got to grips with them about why I was going to be visiting again. I was just conscious of the fact that I was phoning them up and saying 'How

are you today?' and 'How are the children?' and 'Shall I pop round?'. I think those things are just too trivialising.

Assessment and planning failures were sometimes seen as direct deficiencies of more formal social work skills.

> The assessment I made was very superficial. I just feel it's been very messy. There haven't been clear goals. As far as the family was concerned the goal was to *cure* her... I then felt really at a loss. I don't know whether there is a key, but I didn't feel I had the skills to *unlock* that problem and that it was all surface containment... Basically I feel it's been a very messy affair. The *tangible quality* of life of this client was actually deteriorating.

The complexity of social work skills, lack of purposefulness, and the danger that social work may be making matters *worse* were all included in this social worker's concern.

Being in control and being constructive are two parts of a 'game plan'. More difficult to identify, but nonetheless important, is the third aspect of a game plan - staying in the ball park. A probation officer described a pre-sentence report in which a conditional discharge was recommended and where a custodial sentence was given.

> If the judge had said, 'No. Conditional discharge isn't serious enough, I'll fine her', then I'd say, 'fair enough'. I was in the ball park, you know.

An important point is being made. He believed he had been outside the ball park in the sense that he had unwittingly but completely misjudged the rules of the game. The rules may be relatively encompassing but practice is not possible unless the players are on the same turf. We will see later how a practitioner knows the rules when we consider the evidence that social workers believe is sufficient to allow a judgement to be made about good or bad practice.

'It's a bit about knowing your prey'

Having a game plan is a *general* strategy. This general strategy is unlikely to be effective without a strategy specific to the needs of a *particular* individual, group or family - an approach based on knowing the target of intervention - 'knowing your prey'. There were three elements to knowing your prey. They are constant watchfulness and awareness, 'the knowledge', and the possession of good timing.

> Evaluation is something which I do by thinking, by observing, the dialogue with the client, the dialogue with other people I work alongside from other agencies and this agency... You have to be constantly aware.

This watchfulness demands perspective and detachment. As one community worker put it, 'Are you speaking the words or are you looking down at yourself speaking the words?' The knowledge behind a trained eye is essentially personal. 'It sounds a bit non-specific I know, but you do rely on your own life experience, your own experience of parenting... I think I've got the knowledge.' Watchfulness and 'the knowledge' help develop the third element, a sense of *timing*, whether it was the good timing of deciding when to place young children for adoption, or the absence of timing described by the project staff member who picked the wrong moment to breathalyse someone 'and the outcome was to damage our relationship for a couple of months.'

Having a good client

Watchfulness and knowing your prey may be insufficient if the social worker is working with someone they do not regard as a good client. We will tell this aspect of practitioners' stories in the next chapter when considering client evaluations of good practice. For the moment we can simply note that a good client who copes, plans, is able to talk, focuses on the future, and shares key aspects of the practitioner's own approach, is often seen as a key contribution to practice which goes well.

'Just sheer luck'

Whatever personal game plans may be in place, and however experienced and wise a social worker may be, there remains, for the social workers we spoke to, an element of unpredictability close to the heart of social work practice. At its simplest it is reflected in the assumption of one social worker that 'there's always an element of good fortune in these things.'

> Whether it was because the time was right for her and I was just lucky that I connected I don't know. I think it was just sheer luck. It's a bit like gambling and roulette, and every now and then you score the right number and you make a good connection with somebody. It just happened for that client and for me it was the right time.

The commonly expressed view that cases are capable of 'blowing up into a total nightmare' assumes that there are aspects of work that are beyond the control of even the seasoned game-planner. If outcomes are no easier to predict than a number on a roulette wheel, an important conclusion may seem to follow. Social workers cannot be held accountable for work going wrong nor praised for work going well. Indeed, we did not speak to any social workers who took full blame for work which had not gone well. Various reasons were suggested as mitigating factors, and the theme of control was once again prominent, most frequently in the argument that there were aspects that could not be expected to lie within the social worker's control. 'I don't feel I did the piece of work as well as I might have done, but, having said that there were elements in it that were totally out of my control.'

This lack of control sometimes stemmed from the belief that the standards to which the social worker was working were set by others and not owned by the practitioner. 'The reason I'm feeling I've failed is because the expectations were from the funder.' The circumstances of daily work may also mitigate the degree of personal blame. 'The nature of the work here, gets you into that state sometimes...That's one of the traps that we regularly fall into.'

A convincing conclusion from listening to these social workers is that, although they almost always identify substantial mitigating factors when work does not go well - and often decline the credit when work turns out happily - practitioners rarely if ever duck out of all responsibility. Indeed, social workers often set themselves very high standards. 'I think sometimes I beat myself with a stick' could be said by many social workers.

This reference to personal, emotional evidence forms a bridge between how social workers describe their *strategies* for evaluating in practice, and the specific *evidence* they draw on for the work they describe.

Evidence for quality

We have seen the evaluation strategy employed by social workers. It has confirmed our earlier twin conclusions that evaluating does happen, but that it is troublesome or threatened with marginalisation. But what evidence is sufficient to persuade a practitioner that work has gone well or badly? There was a high degree of agreement among people working in diverse agency settings. The perceived quality of their work depended on the answers they obtained to a range of questions.

1.   Does the work produce emotional rewards or penalties for the social worker?

2.   Did the social worker's intervention win steady, incremental change?

3.   Was the case or problem hitherto 'stuck' or 'moving'?

4.   Did the client provide positive feedback within the social work relationship?

5.   Did fellow professionals provide corroborating evidence on the quality of the work?

6.   Has the social work process as such harmed the client?

Emotional rewards and penalties

It might be thought that social workers, weaned knowingly or unknowingly on the heritage of Biestek's principle of controlled emotional involvement, would at least be wary of admitting the emotional impact of the work they do, and even more so of giving it a central place in reaching decisions about how well their work was going. Far from it. Barely any of the people we spoke to failed to locate the evidence of the emotions as central to their direct practice evaluating. Even the rare sceptic admitted as much.

> There was a certain amount of gut feeling on my part as to how it was going. Which I think is quite a problem when you come to evaluating. How can you separate your gut feeling from what's actually happening?

'Quite a comfort', 'excites', 'enjoy', 'flattering', 'reassuring', 'a brilliant experience for me', 'a sense of satisfaction', 'real pleasure', 'a good feeling', 'on form' - these are just a scattering of the phrases that came immediately to people's minds when they were asked how they knew they were doing well in particular instances. The recognition that good feelings were not common only served to make these emotional responses more appreciated.

> It makes a change. I mean we don't often get real pleasure in child protection work. Is it important? Yeah, a sense that something good has come out of the work that we've done. Yes, I think that is important.

There is sometimes an unpredictable immediacy to the emotional rewards. It was this feature that led to social workers talking about 'luck' in their work. A community worker described a group that took off unexpectedly after three or four years as follows.

> The buzz was there. People wanted to work. I was on form. The other thing it was a one off... The buzz was there, people were involved, everybody was talking, everybody felt safe.

We have seen already that 'gut feeling' was appealed to as a basis for knowing that a particular piece of practice was outside the ball park. Emotional reactions were evidence of practice going badly just as they were confirmation of it going well. 'I'm getting absolutely *nowhere* with her, and so it makes me feel quite frustrated...I don't get any sense of satisfaction in any of the interactions I have with her.'

The influence of the emotions on practice sometimes led to inappropriate moral judgements, and to a worry that good practice could thus be put at risk. 'My frustrations show when I'm with her and that's not helpful - to her, to the kids, or to me.' Social work's emotional reward system operates both ways. 'I wasn't getting anything out of the relationship, and she wasn't getting anything out of the probation order.'

Client change

Emotional payoffs are crucial parts of the jigsaw of evidence but they are not all. 'You want the sessions to be fun but you want them to be effective as well'. Change matters, and the client's 'movement' was seen as a vital clue to this having occurred. Behaviour change and attitude change were the two indicators.

> The relationship with the mother is much better, the bedwetting's improved, school situation's been sorted out, offending and truanting's stopped. So those were the practical things that indicated to me that things were successful, and also there's the boy and his mother's words and attitudes.

Social workers rarely made any distinction between *outputs* - the products which may or may not have anything to do with the intervention - and direct *outcomes*. When asked if the same results would have occurred if the social worker had not been involved, most were fairly confident that clients would not have reached a positive destination without the social worker's attentions, or if so, they would have taken much longer about it. But one or two were less sure.

> When you're dealing with people's lives, it's difficult to know whether your intervention causes anything to happen or whether it would have happened anyway.

'One step at a time'

We have already noticed the value that social workers place on the achievement of small, incremental goals as part of their strategy, and this was reflected in the evidence they cited.

> I started off wanting to have an effect on his *offending*, bringing in something to reduce the anxiety that *led* to the offending and so on and so forth. I found really quite quickly that all those were far, far too grand and ambitious and he really wasn't interested in any of them. So I thought, well, if nothing else, you can at least keep him company once a week.

Just as grand goals were eschewed, so a social worker could explain why she was not happy with the standards she had been using in a piece of work that had gone badly. She needed 'more of a sense of *realism*. I got sucked into the idea of thinking that this is a situation that can be *cured*.' Achieving incremental change was positive evidence for good practice, as when a probation officer described his work with a shoplifter in uncompromising, self-effacing terms.

> I suppose I've felt on more than one occasion that something was hitting home a little bit and I was maybe chipping away at some of her assumptions...

> The fact that I can successfully get her to begin to think about something which might in the end turn a few little cogs in her mind is gonna be for her a success. If there is only a little, *tweeny* chink in the wall of justification for offending, then, yeah, I would probably take a little bit of credit for that.

In another practitioner's words, 'at the end we'd reached all the goals that were set. They weren't *big* ones, but we'd reached all of them.' Most social workers would be more than happy with steady, step-by-step change of this kind.

'Stuck' or 'moving'?

Evidence of good practice was all the more persuasive if it was achieved in the context of problems which hitherto had been 'stuck'. We saw earlier the example of the community worker who had been working with a group 'for ages now, and I've been trying to help them to get some sort of plan for three or four years.' Similarly, a probation officer described his long-term shoplifter case who 'was given to me as 'Oh your turn, everyone else has had a crack. Your turn to take her on'.

> I felt it was quite important because she'd been on probation so *many* times and really had talked about anything and everything. Probation officers had pretty much done it all before. Weighed up against other clients...I thought of her rather than them as a success because the task was always going to be *massively* more difficult to start off with.

Gaining confirmation

Gaining some corroboration that work had gone well was often mentioned by social workers. Interestingly, however, direct feedback from clients was rarely given as evidence. When it did come, it was a rare red letter day. 'I'd be a *liar* if I said that wasn't important to me.' The corroboration of fellow professionals was, however, mentioned far more frequently. Explaining why he knew a piece of work had gone well, a social worker said,

> from the dialogue I have with the other professionals in the case. We all tend to agree upon the same issues. We don't necessarily agree on how to resolve them but we all agree what those issues are.

The probation officer who had ended up with a recommendation for a conditional discharge being turned into a custodial sentence believed that the failure of professional corroboration was a central problem.

> The court officer who'd seen the report before it went into court was as shocked as I was, and the person who 'gate-kept' the report was equally shocked, and we were all absolutely stunned.

When professional collaboration did break down, it could feel close to a major disaster. Speaking of a situation that had gone very badly wrong, a social worker explained how she had written a confidential and frank letter about a client which had been read out in a case conference. 'I just felt totally betrayed, ridiculed and humiliated by the whole experience to be honest with you....and everybody I felt thought "What a bitch of a social worker".'

To do no harm

A core concern among social workers was their need to reach a judgement about whether the system of social service provision had avoided making matters still worse for the client and other service users. Work that had gone well was often evidenced on the grounds that no harm had been done when there seemed reason to fear it might. Evidence that work had not gone well was often presented in terms of the damaging impact of the welfare system. Social workers were not so much concerned at this point with whether social work had achieved any demonstrable impact, but with whether the process of service delivery had been accomplished with integrity. After describing a very complex family situation, a child protection social worker concluded,

> the most important thing at the end of the day is that two little boys who could've been *lost* within a system that sometimes takes *far too long*, they're not lost, they are two very happy, confident, loved little boys.

Work that goes badly is often regarded as having exacerbated the service user's problems.

> We weren't able as a centre to keep confidentiality. Everybody got involved so it was a real mess. When I look back there was no need to involve so many people, everybody in the centre to know her business. I can't imagine how that woman felt about everybody knowing what was going on in her life. I think she felt intimidated.

Perhaps the most reflective account was given by a member of a duty team, who tellingly illustrated how personal evaluation methods can form a coherent strategy based on humanising the system.

> Whether I've made it a little bit easier to understand for people, whether I've made the pathway through it a little bit easier and a little bit less stressful, whether I've given them sufficient information, whether I've made it a little bit less dramatic, a little bit easier to pick up the threads afterwards.

Thus in the work that had gone well she concluded 'I haven't alienated this lady...I think she was able to grasp that she was an important part of this whole problem and she wasn't just someone being forgotten about'. Conversely, in the work that had not gone well - a call-out to a man being held at a police station for an assessment under the Mental Health Act - the social worker explained that the problem did not lie in the *outcome* but in the *process*. 'We've admitted somebody correctly, but I still don't think I did it very well.'

Accounts of evaluating

Much of the evaluating in action described by these practitioners is without doubt good practice. The work is described in an informed and persuasive tone, and the issues raised by these narratives echo loudly through subsequent chapters. This evidence, together with the small amount of recent research dealing with evaluating practice, helps to sharpen a number of questions.

Accounts and accountability

Poor practice is likely to trigger deep uncertainties in the mind of the reflective social worker. Am I responsible? Should I take the blame? Could it have been avoided? The social worker whose candid letter about a client had been read out in a case conference puzzled over her accountability as follows.

> I do feel on my part that was bad practice, personally you know, because I just felt had I known ...But then I don't know. I suppose it's a *bit* of blame on my part, and I think that possibly in the future I wouldn't divulge stuff like that, and whether that would be good or bad I don't know. Probably bad... So I don't know whether it's my fault. I don't think it is (my fault) because I've been monitoring the case, not in the way I should be monitoring it, which is bad I feel... I feel I totally failed there and the sad thing is I've still got her. I mean that's the sad thing for me, you know. Where do we go now? I don't know.

The dilemma is unforgivingly sharp. There are two realities that need to be brought into conjunction.

First, there is a widespread sense that outcomes, both good and bad, are beyond prediction and will never cease to jump out and surprise the practitioner. Social workers - at least the ones we spoke to - are characterised by this uncertainty. Second, social workers display a hesitation about claiming credit for good work or blame for bad work. We have suggested some possible reasons for this, including the perceived complexity of social work, competing interests, and the private nature of much social work practice which is not visible to colleagues.

The two realities - predicting and accountability - are linked. Consider the probation officer who recommended a conditional discharge for a woman who then received a four-month custodial sentence. The probation officer's response was that this is an 'understandable' error. With hindsight he thought that he could have found out that passing a forged note even for a small sum would be treated seriously; 'but even then it still wouldn't strike me as a serious offence', because the incident was difficult to anticipate and was essentially unpredictable.

> Whether that constitutes a failure it's so difficult to assess because there's so many variables...you can't predict. You could have a great report and a dodgy defence solicitor, you could have a dodgy report and a great defence solicitor, and have the same outcome.

Finally, as we have seen earlier, he pointed to the way he had used all the expected avenues of advice and consultation, and the system had failed to flag up the potential hazard. The conclusion seemed to him inescapable.

> I think, bearing in mind the fact that you can't predict what judges are going to do, you can't predict what magistrates are going to do, in a sense you can't take the blame for a failure. If you can't take the blame if it doesn't work, how can you take the credit if it does?

Humphrey and Pease similarly discovered among probation officers a belief that there is an element of luck in being effective, and that you could do brilliant work but if the circumstances are against you then the outcome will be poor. 'If luck is seen to determine outcome, probation supervision becomes merely a matter of keeping an offender in the community for luck to strike' (Humphrey and Pease, 1992: 36). As a consequence clients may get into further trouble but probation officers did not think such further offending reflected in any way on the quality of their practice. An American study of social workers in private social work practice heard social workers acknowledging that, just as poor outcomes are not the responsibility of the practitioner, so 'it's hard to take credit in this sort of work for really helping people' (Elks and Kirkhart, 1993: 556).

Causes and accounts

We have seen that in their day-to-day work social workers do not give formal cause-and-effect explanations of events.   They are more concerned with rules, conventions and the meaning of their work, on the one hand, and with uncertainty and approximations to knowledge on the other.   A number of writers have reasoned that as a consequence

> Rule following, convention obeying, meaning giving or any other form of self monitoring is fatal to the idea that the heart of an explanation lies in the causal story
>
> (Harré and Secord, 1972: 168).

Rule governed behaviour is 'not to do with the inevitability of causal necessity but with the inexorability of moral necessity' (Harré, 1989: 35).   Should we conclude from this that causal explanations form at the most a marginal and insignificant part of social work practice?   An exploration of the character of 'case talk' between social workers in a children's team reached the conclusion that such talk takes on a dramatic narrative character in which causal accounts are marginal.   Case presentations to line managers take the form of a moral tale, in which the responsibility of any failure is typically ascribed to the client rather than the social worker, where there is little explicit theorising, and in which the behaviour is not related to specific causes but is part of the narrative drama.

> The experienced worker, through soundings, brief forays and insightful observations of family relations, can construct a mosaic of suspicions that confirms the presence of 'problems' without specifying the precise cause or cure...The construction of a 'case' is thus a *rhetorical* accomplishment
>
> (Pithouse and Atkinson, 1988: 197).

Yet although rhetoric and moral persuasion are a crucial aspect of daily practice, social workers also regard themselves as working towards a knowledge of cases which will serve as a good enough approximation to identifiable personal or social problems.   Incomplete and maybe flawed causal understandings are an ingredient of these explanations.   'People do have strong intuitions concerning the presence or absence of causes in particular instances' and it is probable that 'systematic rules and strategies' exist 'for assessing cause in...everyday inference' (Einhorn and Hogarth, 1986: 3). Although it inevitably has fuzzy boundaries, the concept of cause is a viable one if only because we continue to function well enough in terms of it. While social workers may not appeal to causes in a formal sense, they are centrally concerned with giving explanations and reasons (Draper, 1988).

People engage in causal reasoning in order to make sense of the world. It is therefore likely to be unusual or abnormal events that arouse causal interest, and such explanations are of central importance if we are to understand how social workers explain and account for things going wrong or even unusually well. We can identify four different kinds of account (Lyman and Scott, 1970; Bull and Shaw, 1992).

> *Excuses* are offered when someone accepts that an action is bad, wrong or inappropriate, but responsibility is denied.

> *Confessions* are made when both responsibility and blame are accepted.

> *Justifications* take the form of accepting responsibility, but denying the pejorative quality of the action.

> *Repudiations* reject both blame and responsibility for an action.

Social worker accounts of work that is going well or not are both attempts to explain a problem and a professional safety net. For example, a causal account may secure colleague and management approval for limited achievement in the past and in the future. Social workers offer both *retrospective* and *prospective* justifications for limited and imprecise effects from social work intervention, and for an incremental style of work described by one respondent as 'chipping away'.

We have seen that in constructing these explanations social workers engage in a kind of 'lay theorising' (Furnham, 1988). We are not attempting to justify untidy thinking and practice, but rather to warn against viewing social workers' alleged lack of formal rationality as an immature primitivism. Such crudely positivist - I intend this as a swear word - ethnocentrism will not suffice. A perspective which accepts that social workers are engaged in giving and making accounts requires us to recognise that social work practice is more complex than we often allow. Finding a persuasive causal account to justify or excuse things that go wrong will always be at the heart of social workers' evaluating in practice competencies.

Complex and ambiguous evidence

Social workers' uncertainties are also strengthened by their conviction that evidence will always prove more or less ambiguous and complex, and open to competing interpretations. 'I personally don't feel a hundred per cent certain about anything I do. I think its so difficult when you're working with individuals.'

Evidence is occasionally straightforward. For social workers operating in a project or residential setting a wrong move may lead to a more or less instant reaction. 'You're often very conscious of handling things wrong and developing bad practice when you get immediate payback.' However, 'immediate payback' is not the usual state of affairs. Employing an apt simile one social worker concluded,

> It's like snap photographs - one individual photograph isn't going to tell you very much. Over a period of time, that's how we see things, but that's not easy.

We have already heard several examples of chastened social workers relating stories of how they had felt 'taken in' by clients, partly because of the ambiguity of evidence. Probation officers were almost unanimous in drawing attention to this aspect of their work.

> I'm a bit angry with myself because part of me should have...been a little less willing to flatter myself - to be as easily drawn along as I was. On paper for the first year it looked a brilliant piece of work. I mean it was all planned out, supervision plans and it looked great. And it was actually a piece of work I was proud of until that point. But built on sand - it was myth.

This picture receives support from a study of social workers dealing with child sexual abusers, where social workers trod a fine line between listening to the perpetrators' accounts and avoiding being manipulated by their rationalisations. One social worker in this study said,

> Every gesture, every word, every moment that I've got contact with the sex offender, I'm working really hard to keep myself in some sort of balance, not having it distorted or manipulated, and it's very subtle'
> (Waterhouse, Dobash and Carnie, 1995: 152).

It is inevitable that ambiguity will be ever present. 'Sincerity was difficult to gauge and there were no guarantees the 'correct' responses offered by the abuser were genuinely held.' In consequence there is an endemic uncertainty which social workers have to live with. 'How can professionals know if their intervention is having any effect on perpetrators. How are they to ascertain if progress is being made? The short and immediate answer from those directly involved was that they can never be sure' (pp 160, 170).

Knowing and feeling

We have encountered an apparent paradox in practitioners' narratives. Luck, cloudy accountability, complex evidence and inherently uncertain outcomes all appear to imply that practitioners are unlikely to feel confident about the value and impact of their work. Yet social workers often appear confident they know what they are doing. There is an assumed knowledge, a tacit understanding that is based on having a 'game plan', knowing your targets and a reliance on proven 'gut feeling'. A prison psychiatrist remarked to Waterhouse and her colleagues, 'It's a sort of intangible thing. It's a feeling you get that somebody's being genuine; sometimes it rings true and sometimes it doesn't' (p161). A social worker in the same project said of sexual abuse perpetrators, 'you begin to get an instinct for them, when he's being honest and when he isn't' (p171).

The social workers we spoke to called heavily on their own emotional reactions to practice, alongside their 'gut feeling'. Social work is an occupation that entails 'emotional labour', 'the management of feeling to create a publicly observable facial and bodily display.' 'Filigreed patterns of feeling and their management' (Hochschild, 1983: 7, 11) make up the emotional style of social work. Social workers run with a tension between a training and agency culture which cultivates a 'managed heart', and an enriching utilisation of the evidence of their emotions as they evaluate their day-to-day work. They would probably agree with Erikson that the clinician's own feelings and opinions are an essential ingredient of clinical inference.

> The evidence is not 'all in' if he does not succeed in using his own emotional responses during a clinical encounter as an evidential source and as a guide to intervention'
>
> (Erikson, 1959: 93).

We have considered at some length in this chapter how social workers handle the complex question of knowing whether they are doing well in their practice. We have observed the two very different models of evaluation held by practitioners, and the specific strategies they adopt to evaluate in daily practice. In the latter part of this book we argue for evaluating in practice competencies that take seriously these realities of present practice. In the next chapter we explore social workers' beliefs about how clients and carers evaluate services, and listen to their inspections of how far they thought service users were in tune with their own practice evaluations.

4   The evaluating client

He doesn't like being examined: it's too close to an evaluation, which is too close to a judgement. If there are judgements going around he wants to be making them himself.

Margaret Atwood ('Robber Bride')

The boys would have said they enjoyed it, and they would probably say it made them think. They would probably have less faith in its effectiveness than I did. A few of them were quite critical. 'Yeah, well it's fine you can sit and talk about those things in here, but it's not like that out in the real world.

Probation Officer

Social work has oscillated between celebration and mistrust of client accounts. For a combination of reasons which make uneasy bedfellows, celebration is presently in the ascendant. This acclaim presents us with a range of questions. What benefits stem from studies of service users' evaluations of practice? What frameworks do clients and carers operate within when evaluating social work? How do practitioners perceive the relationship between their own evaluations and those of clients? Is partnership in evaluating between social workers and clients likely to be straightforward or will it face special difficulties? Is 'consumer satisfaction' the yardstick against which social work practice must be measured? These questions provide the agenda for this chapter.

Client evaluations of social work

It is difficult to think ourselves back to the period of social work practice before the publication of Mayer and Timms' *The Client Speaks*, which triggered a steady stream of research that changed practitioners' basic assumptions regarding the significance of service users' knowledge, belief and attitudes regarding the social work practice offered to them.

In his review of the implications of this research for practice, Howe concludes that 'clients consistently say similar kinds of things about their experiences of being helped (and not being helped), no matter what school of counselling they have attended' (Howe, 1993: 1). In doing so, clients appear to be identifying general, non-specific, processes and experiences that cut across different schools of intervention. Should we draw the conclusion that 'It is not the specific technique that is important but the manner in which it is done and the way it is experienced (p3)? Howe's interpretation goes an important step further than this. He illustrates in some detail that these non-specific conditions are valued by service users because they provide a vehicle within which talk and dialogue can take place. Methods of intervention, therefore, *do* matter. They provide the non-specific context for seeking to make sense of problems through talk. Accept me, understand me and talk with me are the three practice injunctions which Howe believes follow from the steady build-up over the last two or three decades of our knowledge of what takes place within social work.

Should we conclude from this that there is essentially a fundamental harmony between clients and carers when it comes to picturing what is going on within social work? Probably not. It is unhelpful to assume that there is a global 'client's experience' or 'carer's experience'. Gender, disability, age and generational factors, race and agency differences will all cross-cut the common status of being a service user. Likewise, there are significant differences between the experience of 'captive' clients, non-captive clients and carers (Sainsbury, Nixon and Phillips, 1982; Fisher, 1992). For example, we now know something about the distinctive experience of parents, older people, children, black service users, and people with learning disabilities or mental health problems (Fisher and Marsh, 1986; Barnes, 1992; Barnes and Wistow, 1994; Butler and Williamson, 1994; Beresford, 1992; Pitcairn, 1994; Whittaker, 1994; Ahmed, 1989; Fisher, Newton and Sainsbury, 1984).

We have stressed likely service user differences in how they experience social work, but this should not allow us to fragment that experience.   Ways in which the experience of service users has a common core are illustrated from research carried out with children entering and leaving care. When seeking to understand how families understood the process of entering care, the researchers assumed 'care' would be viewed by parents as an infringement of their rights because legal custody of their child was no longer theirs. 'It was somewhat surprising therefore to encounter an extensive lack of concern on the part of the majority of parents over whether care had effected their rights as parents. The sense of infringement was denied or the topic was seen as irrelevant' (Fisher, Marsh and Phillips, 1986: 56).

The parents' main concern was a quite different one, and sprang from the conviction that they held a *moral* responsibility and right to 'teach them right from wrong' - the right to retain a say about pocket money, going to bed, bad language, friends and so on. For these parents entry into care was not an *abrogation* of rights but a consonant *expression* of their rights by acting 'for their own good'. It was itself an *exercise* of responsibility rather than merely a *transfer*. Therefore parents' expectations of care centred around authority and discipline. They wanted reassurance as to whether the person doing the caring shared their own attitude to responsibility, and exercised it according to what they believed their child needed.

Later work has confirmed this conclusion that parents are likely to think in terms of moral sanctions rather than legal ones (Fisher, 1983). This difference between social workers and parents may, of course, lead to social workers concentrating carefully on issues of legal rights, and 'sensitively handling topics which were not uppermost in parents' minds' (Fisher, Marsh and Phillips, 1986: 62). While this research is about children who become subject to statutory intervention, it is probable that other service users who are 'captive' clients and carers will share a common meaning and experience.

Recent work on understanding personal experience through narrative offers a promising approach to developing a shared evaluation of practice which nonetheless steers away from assuming that social workers and client accounts can easily be merged. The oscillation we have noted between mistrust and confidence in client accounts is due in part to debates over the exact status of such accounts. Are they pictures of how the world really is, or are they essentially claims constructed in the process of social work?   The attraction of client studies lies partly in the belief that the accounts they produce are in important ways more 'true' than welfare professionals' accounts.

Advocates of narrative inquiry approaches would conclude that,

> Story is...neither raw sensation nor cultural form; it is both and neither. In effect, stories are the closest we can come to experience as we and others tell our experience...

> Experience, in this view, is the stories people live. People live stories, and in the telling of them reaffirm them, modify them, and create new ones.
> (Clandinin and Connelly, 1994:415).

When hearing the client we need to distinguish the client's story, the telling of the story, the life experience of people in the story, our experience of the story, and the wider audience of people who read our text or account. In consequence, the social worker operates 'in a forest of events and stories pointing inward and outward, and backward and forward' (p418).

This approach underscores several important considerations. First, the relation between telling the story and living the story are inextricably intertwined. 'People are both living their stories...and telling their stories in words as they reflect upon life and explain themselves to others' (Connelly and Clandinin, 1990: 4). In addition, the story is shaped by the telling. To tell the story is to 'restory' it. 'It is a hard thing to make up stories to live by' (Heilbrun, cited by Connelly and Clandinin, p2).

Narrative inquiry perspectives also presume that clients and social workers are both engaged in narrative work. It is not a case of social workers listening to, recording, appraising and 'using' client accounts. Just as clients are story tellers and story livers, so likewise are social workers. They are not scribes. The ways in which practice should be influenced by such accounts is a matter to which we return on several occasions during this book. But all participants have 'voice' and have to play a believing game which involves inserting oneself in the other's story as a way of coming to know the other's story and giving voice to the other.

Service users and practitioners

At this point in the chapter we pick up again the stories and accounts of social workers as they talk about examples of work which they thought went either particularly well or less well. In what respects do practitioners think their own service delivery is informed by knowing the judgements and evaluations made by those on the receiving end of services? Do social workers think that clients' and carers' methods of evaluating are akin to or different from their own?

We do not know, of course, whether the views ascribed to clients by social workers would be accepted by those clients were we in a position to ask them. Our focus is instead on what social workers believed to be the case. Do social workers believe they are in agreement with service users in their evaluations of service delivery? How feasible is such agreement? Do social workers rate these questions as important? Important, that is, not in the general and relatively detached sense of whether they think partnership with clients is a good thing, or believe that clients have the right to be listened to, but in the more immediate sense of whether they believe they give weight to such matters in their day-to-day practice? These apparently honest accounts provide, as we have said already, the essential empirical connections for developing an evaluating in practice that makes sense of the real contexts of daily practice.

Social workers' answers to these questions fell into four main groups. First, some social workers thought that clients shared their view about the overall direction of the outcome, and also that they based their judgements on similar considerations and premises to those held by the practitioner. Second, a number of social workers thought that clients and those close to them did not share either the general direction of the assessment or the criteria on which it was based. This was particularly so when practitioners were considering occasions where the work had gone less well.

A third and larger group of social workers found the question more difficult to answer. Although the service users would in the social workers' view agree that it went well or not, they would have used different criteria. Finally, there were occasions when the social worker either did not know the client's view or thought that the issue was one the client had not considered. A few social workers argued that the whole question did not and could not make sense to the people with whom they had been working. We will illustrate each of these responses, and consider their implications for partnership in evaluating between practitioner and client.

Agreeing and disagreeing

The first group of social workers included two instances where all had gone well. The work led to a good result, the service user agreed, and everyone appeared to be working to a shared agenda. It is a demanding level of agreement and it was only apparent on these two occasions. As one of them put it,

> I don't think it's true of many cases but in this particular case I think they would agree. A lot of the work that we did was centred around whose needs were going to be met first. And it was the children. And one of the things she was saying was 'I don't want my children to end up like I am'.

Mutual agreement about evaluations was equally apparent in those instances where, even though the work itself had not gone well, the practitioner and the client or carers had achieved consensus on that point. This also happened in two instances. For example, having decided he was engaged in pointless and potentially damaging visits to a family, a child protection social worker concluded,

> I think the client was glad we actually nailed it down. She really was talking about herself in a way which I would have looked at as well. Yeah, she was looking at it in much the same way as how I expect most social workers would look at it.

On the contrary, there were a number of practice examples where clear water existed between the social worker's evaluation and what they believed to be the client's evaluation. For example, one social worker thought a case had gone very well where the client had been removed from a residential unit, and was now living independently. However,

> the family were really annoyed when we terminated the placement...You get a lot of families that like their relatives to respond the way they've always responded, in other words controlled by them...I could imagine that the family probably see that as something very awful because they've no longer got control over their little girl.

More common were disagreements of the kind where the social worker thought the work had not gone well, but the client or those close to them, took a contrary and positive view.

> He would probably tell you that it had been very helpful. He basically stuck by his thing that the work we had done in that first year was genuine. That's

one of the things I actually did do...talk to him about what value it has been, because I don't think we've really touched base on what's been happening, and he's countered that by saying, No, he found it helpful.

I think he'd probably say 'Oh, he's quite a nice bloke, he's friendly, and he's polite and he talks to me tidy. He's helped me sort out getting a flat and he gave me an electricity token today. He made me pay him back but he got it for me.' I think he'd be reasonably positive about it.

Different priorities

The second and third groups of social workers thought that consensus between them and service users was partial, more apparent than real, or based on a different agenda. These accounted for about half of the instances of work that social workers discussed with us. For example, members of the family might agree that things had not gone well, but would, in the social worker's eyes, be viewing issues from a different viewpoint. We saw in the previous chapter that social workers tended to eschew grand goals. One of the most common reasons for unshared evaluation priorities between practitioners and service users was when inappropriately ambitious goals were believed to be held by clients and families.

Oh, they wouldn't see my role as being effective at all. Not unless I can get her a new house tomorrow. The mum, where she sees effectiveness, is quite different to where I see effectiveness is.

They want some kind of pill that she can take and make it all better. As far as their daughter is concerned it was either cure or nothing.

More interesting, perhaps, were those cases where social worker and client both apparently thought that the work went well, but where the social workers were convinced that subtle but important divergence existed on priorities. Probation officers tended to think that, even if things had gone well, clients were less likely to rate the reduction of offending as the first priority. Speaking about the outcome of a group for offenders one officer said,

She'd probably say, 'Yeah, it's all right' in a sense that I got a couple of things for her. I wrote a couple of letters so that she didn't have to come into town to get her dole cheque. She'd probably say I've been reasonably understanding, that I gave her the benefit of the doubt. I can't imagine her speaking highly of the fact that I pressed her on exactly why she shoplifted. I don't think she'd be terribly impressed by that.

Social workers tended to explain divergent priorities in terms of clients being more preoccupied with their personal wellbeing than the social worker would have preferred. A community worker, reflecting on the successful planning stages for a Black women's information and self-help group, concluded,

> I think they would be quite happy, because it's something they've been asking for, the opportunity to be with other women, the children will be looked after in the creche, it will be like a day out for them, taking them out of the house. But I think they will see the information being not as important as I see it. 'We'll be out of the house, we'll have a nice lunch, the kids will be looked after, we'll be together.' I think that would be the list of priorities for them.

The context of these reservations is important, because they were both examples of good and successful work. In other words, good and successful work, even when practitioner and service user agree, does not necessarily mean that agreement over goals was achieved. Likewise with the following,

> He had a very simple goal and he's achieved it. He wanted to move. He never really admitted that his behaviour was a problem. For him what mattered was his unhappiness and he didn't really care what the consequences were for anybody else. And I don't think he'd particularly see that as being a consequence of my work. The benefits in terms of improved behaviour are external ones that I see and the rest of the staff.

The social worker reasoned similarly for the family involved in this same case.

> The family member with whom he was living, to be honest, is glad to be shot of him, so in a sense I think he's probably achieved his goal as well, at minimum inconvenience to himself. He just wanted this person removed from the family. Which happened. So he'd probably say it was a very successful outcome.

The frequency with which social workers believe they are working to a different agenda from clients or other service users seems to make the possibility of full partnership in assessment, planning and evaluation improbable.

Asking the right question

The remainder of the people we spoke to either did not know the client's view or thought the question made untenable assumptions. Several social workers thought it was hard to say, or were not really sure that the client had ever thought about it. 'She may not view it in the same light, so that's a very difficult one for me personally, how she would have felt.'

Careful arguments were put forward by two social workers, a child protection social worker and a probation officer, to the effect that the question did not, and probably could not, make sense in some contexts. The child protection social worker argued from the premise that the client is always the child, and not the parent. The client system and the target system are always separate. Therefore, in situations where a voluntary partnership does not prove feasible, 'the service user may not have a say in the matter.' To these social workers, it becomes irrelevant in one sense whether or not the service user thinks the work has gone well. Judgement has to be made on the grounds of evidence that the child is safe and free from significant harm and that needs are being met.

An argument to the same effect was put forward by a probation officer working in a court setting.

> Clients always do have a different agenda, because when you interview a client their first feeling is, 'right, you're here to help them.'

But more importantly, practitioners believe that clients in this setting are unlikely to ask themselves whether they have received a good service. 'I think she hasn't probably even thought about it.' Indeed, the client *cannot* ask the question because of the nature of the system.

> I don't think she'll have the insight into the role of the report, or even the way it was written, to even consider whether there was a problem...What effect the report had on the process is probably too far divorced from what happened for her to worry about whether the service she got was satisfactory or not.

Consequently clients do not possess any 'rules' of good practice. This probation officer was embarrassed by the family's telephone call of thanks when a custodial sentence had been passed. To the probation officer this was 'a bizarre thing to do', just because it fell outside any rules for the appreciation of service standards.

Not only do clients have no set of rules to judge service, they do not have any control over the process.

> It's just part of the process that people don't control. From the moment they're arrested to the moment they're sentenced they're being dragged from pillar to post by the courts.
>
> The report is just a part of this whole process of going through the system and not really understanding what it's all about but knowing at the end of it you're going to be sentenced, and everything else is irrelevant. It's just a series of, I mean it's disempowering...by the nature of it.

The assumption is persuasive. To be able to evaluate, a service user needs to have some degree of influence and 'voice' about the outcome of their involvement with the agency. Without this voice client evaluation is meaningless. We have more to say about this problem below, but it is hard to dissent from the conclusion drawn from studies of patient satisfaction, that 'the concept of satisfaction can only be meaningful and useful...if service users think, act and evaluate in terms of it.' Yet the conclusion that Williams drew from his wide ranging review was that 'patients often do not evaluate in terms of being satisfied' (Williams, 1994: 514).

Evaluating in partnership?

These accounts raise the question whether a partnership between practitioner and client is feasible in evaluating practice. A probation officer welcomed the recent shifts towards a performance culture on the grounds that 'you have to keep looking at your own practice all the time and look at your practice with the client, so that they feel part of it.' Similar remarks were made about the advent of Community Care packages. 'From that point of view evaluation is quite positive and clients can see the use of it.' A community worker offered a corresponding argument.

> If you build up a trust you can evaluate together. Unless it's a partnership, unless all parties are wanting the same thing from the evaluation then I don't think it'll get acted on.

However, examples of partnership in evaluating are, on the evidence we have seen, very unusual, although when they do happen they are highly valued by the social worker. The extent to which a partnership is likely to occur depends partly on social workers' prior judgements about whether someone is a 'positive client'. When they were identifying evidence to support conclusions that work had gone well, some social workers appealed to the way the client had responded to the intervention.

> The client was positive and wanted to find other things to do instead of offending, so there was more of a rapport...They were goals that were set by both of us...he was the one that was coming up with them...He was motivated to improve...he was part of the working agreement...he was the one who was keen to assess what was happening...Because we had a positive client, we go along with the client.

Corresponding hallmarks of a good client - coping, planning, being able to talk, sharing aspects of the practitioner's own approach, focusing on the future, not the past, and being outward looking in caring for her children - were also specified by a child protection social worker.

> She was coping with the bereavement, trying to contemplate being a single parent...she was able to talk about the kind of support she would have...she was beginning to plan...she was talking about her deceased husband in quite a healthy way. She was clearly projecting into the future rather than dwelling in the past. So really she was measuring herself in a way which I would have looked at as well.

Strategies for fostering collaborative evaluation by service users and practitioners are suggested later in the book. However, the extent to which partnership in evaluating is feasible will be limited if social workers and clients do not share compatible aims and priorities. A sharply defined illustration of this problem is given in the study by Waterhouse, Dobash and Carnie of child sexual abusers. Interviewed following imprisonment, the perpetrators of abuse did not share with social workers and other professionals the view that their behaviour and the harm caused to children should be the central concern. The men did not want to be challenged about their offences, but preferred an answer that located the problem in social or biological circumstances that were outside their control. Reluctant to own or take responsibility for their behaviour, they wanted social workers to assist them in achieving reconciliation over a short space of time with the abuser and the family. As a consequence, even when men were willing to discuss their offences 'the motivation for frankness is varied' (Waterhouse, Dobash and Carnie, 1995: 181).

A fundamental reason for the clash between social workers and child sexual abusers was the strong child-centred agenda behind much of the work with offenders. One offender complained that, 'All they're interested in is the protection of the children; they're not interested in you, not interested in helping you' (p199). The researchers concluded pessimistically that, 'Diverging goals and conflicting perspectives on the appropriate way to deal with those who sexually abuse children will continue to constitute the context for exchanges between social workers and offenders' (p199).

Does this mean that social workers cannot rely on service user evaluations in circumstances where client self-interest is prominent? The question and, of course, the answer, are less obvious than this implies for several reasons.   While the client's interpretations may not necessarily include accurate descriptions of the help they are being offered, they are important as indicators of service users' accounts of services. For example, Fisher and Marsh, in their study of children in care and their families, distinguished between 'honest' and 'true' accounts of their experience of services (Fisher, Marsh and Phillips, 1986). Social workers and clients are both living their stories and telling their stories as they explain themselves to others. The plausibility of such narratives is no more or less problematic for clients than for social workers.

Indeed, there is evidence that client judgements may in some circumstances by more accurate than social workers' (Sainsbury, 1975). For example, just as chronic patients become 'experts' who are more knowledgeable than some medical staff (Carr-Hill, 1992), so experienced, long-standing service users will learn their way round systems of practice provision. Members of consumer associations and carer groups will also develop extensive specialist expertise.

Consumer satisfaction

There is a further reason why service user evaluations cannot be ignored. They provide a potential measure of that illusive quality - consumer satisfaction. So far we have used the terms client, service user and consumer almost interchangeably. But to say 'user' or 'client' rather than 'consumer' is to express a relevant distinction. There is a strong normative dimension to whatever designation is given to service users. For example, the term 'claimant' - now fallen into disuse - carried a strong assumption of right to service, of a service that is largely financial, and that service delivery should not expect any personal change on the part of the claimant.

The idea of a consumer is best captured by distinguishing it from the term 'customer'. While they are in many respects comparable terms, a customer implies some degree of regular and continuing relationship to a supplier, and is in social work language, a 'user'. A consumer is a more abstract figure in an abstract market (Williams, 1976). Consumers include both clients and carers, actual users and potential users, target systems and client systems. *Consumer* satisfaction is inherently more general and at an aggregate level, unlike *client* satisfaction. Some commentators have been careful to avoid the term (eg Fisher, 1983).

Social workers to whom we spoke were not always confident that they knew the mind of their clients and their carers when it came to taking on board clients' satisfaction or unhappiness with practice. Some were openly uncertain, and several of those who thought they knew the client's mind were tentative. They 'could imagine', thought it 'possible', or 'got the impression' that clients held this or that view about the service they had been giving. In addition, they did not speak as if an absence of agreement was thought by them to be particularly problematic. This lack of agreement was equally apparent in circumstances where work had gone well, as it was when practitioners believed they had been operating at a less-than-effective level.

This picture jars with the frequently expressed exhortation from managers, academics and policy makers that consumer satisfaction should occupy centre stage in service assessments. Heralded by the early work of Mayer and Timms, the emergence of consumer research in social work from the late sixties in Britain and America was due to several factors. From the middle of the 1960's social workers became less likely to regard working class culture as impoverishing for individual and family life. The increasing exposure to a burgeoning sociology as part of social work training heightened social workers' awareness of structural disadvantage, and made them mistrustful of any claims that appeared to reinforce professional hegemonies. The growing influence of interpretative sociologies made practitioners cautious of scorning the natural attitude, and increasingly willing to question the assumption that there was only one standard of rationality to apply to the interpretation of human conduct and behaviour.

Closer to home, these developments were associated with a decline of treatment ideologies in social work. Psychodynamic models in particular were regarded as marked by an unhelpful preoccupation with the relatively hidden causes of behaviour, rather than with behaviour as such, and thus leading to an aversion from the client's own assessment of the significance of problematic situations. Consumer studies, with their acceptance of lay, common sense explanations, were part of a reaction against medical models, and evidence of a greater interest in what people do, rather than what they are. Strengthened by a backlash against experimental research studies in social work, which appeared to show that nothing works, consumer satisfaction studies turned the focus of research, temporarily at least, away from outcomes and towards the process of service delivery.

Organisational restructuring has been closely associated with client studies. The Fabian critique of welfare service reforms in the late 1960's (eg Sinfield, 1969) and the creation of Social Services Departments in England and Wales in 1970, helped from different starting points to pave the way both for a move towards a model of service delivery in which clients became consumers (Fisher, 1983), and for the spate of consumer studies in the 1970s. From the close of the following decade, the launch of the Citizen's Charter, legislative restructuring within the National Health Service, a decentralised performance and quality culture, and the requirement to consult users and carers as part of community care planning, combined to redirect consumer satisfaction surveys away from the largely academic initiatives of the seventies and early eighties and towards new models of quality. These were inspired by managerial and 'excellence' criteria on the one hand and consumerist approaches on the other. Carers and users were now cast as participants with a role to play in defining what questions should be asked, and not simply as respondents to surveys over which they had no influence, and whose results they rarely saw.

The real world is not so clearcut. Consultation with carers and users has been carried out with 'varying degrees of commitment, understanding and sophistication' (Barnes and Wistow, 1994: 77), and the meaning, measurement and utilisation of evidence regarding consumer satisfaction are less straightforward than might appear on the surface. We return to the first problem in the next chapter. Here we will outline the main questions that need answers if evidence about consumer satisfaction is to prove genuinely empowering and create more than a fuzzy blur of warm cosiness.

A question asking, 'How satisfied were you with the social work service?', with ratings from 'very satisfied' to 'very dissatisfied', appears plausible evidence of a commitment to listening to the client. However, part of the problem is that 'satisfaction' is almost certainly not a single dimension that can be tapped through a general question of this kind. The National Consumer Council has developed a set of criteria for consumer service evaluation that is based on a model of service quality as measured by its fitness for purpose. Consumer satisfaction assessed against these criteria is measured according to whether it does what it is supposed to do, what it is not supposed to do, its cost, and what it is like to use (National Consumer Council, 1986). Taken together these questions yield ten general criteria against which a consumer can evaluate a service (Figure 4.1).

1	Does it do what it is supposed to do?	→	*Access*	availability, equity of access
		→	*Choice*	
		→	*Quality*	comprehensive, reliability, speed
		→	*Benefits*	to users, to community
2	What is it like to use?	→	*Information*	to aid awareness or use
		→	*Ease and pleasant-ness of use*	
		→	*Representation*	channels to communicate views
3	What does it cost?	→	*Economy and Efficiency*	to citizen, to user
4	Does it do what it is not supposed to do?	→	*Redress*	a complaints process
		→	*Risk*	environment, personal safety

Figure 4.1   Consumer criteria for service evaluation
(Based on National Consumer Council, 1986)

An important drawback of consumer rights models developed in the commercial sector or, as in this case, through the consumer movement, is that they do not easily transfer to the personal social services. However, the National Consumer Council criteria do provide a useful framework which unpacks most possible dimensions of satisfaction and provides a yardstick against which consumer satisfaction measures in social work can be assessed.

Further problems arise, however, when satisfaction questions are asked. There is widespread evidence that satisfaction surveys produce a uniformly high proportion of positive answers. The Barclay committee, in its review of client studies some years ago, found that the average satisfaction level was around 66 per cent, and dissatisfaction rates were running at approximately 20 per cent (Barclay, 1982: 167); and this has proved a uniform, even conservative finding in subsequent reviews of both health and personal social services (Fisher, 1983; Shaw, 1984; Carr-Hill, 1992; Batchelor et al, 1994). In consequence, it has usually not proved feasible to differentiate which service users are more or less likely to be satisfied, and satisfaction surveys often do not tell us what needs to be changed. A strategy which appears at first glance to promise empowerment for service users can too easily prove a prop for conservatism and inaction. The risk is created that 'through high levels of relatively meaningless expressions of satisfaction an illusion of consumerism is created which seldom does anything but endorse the *status quo*' (Williams, 1994: 515). To understand why this is the case, we have to explore what takes place when consumers are asked to evaluate service provision.

We have seen that some of the social workers to whom we spoke argued that clients sometimes cannot ask themselves whether they have received a good service because they do not have any control over the outcomes of their involvement with social workers and probation officers. Without this measure of influence the very idea of evaluation will probably seem alien and meaningless to the client and their carers. If a service is seen as a favour rather than a benefit to which the person is entitled, or as a sanction for offending behaviour, then criticism will be seen as a high risk strategy with no obvious benefits. Power differentials between professionals and service users are too easily ignored by consumerists. The more that people see themselves as powerless, the more likely they are to adjust their aspirations regarding what they can reasonably expect to gain from the exchange. They may come to adopt what Fisher and his colleagues recognised, in their work on the experiences of children cared for by the local authority and their families, as a strong sense of fatalistic resignation - a passive acceptance, especially by mothers, of the loss of parental rights over their children (Fisher, Marsh and Phillips, 1986). In a similar manner, the sick role occupied by hospital patients requires a passivity on their part. In his helpful discussion of whether satisfaction is a valid concept, Williams (1994: 513) has aptly remarked that this passivity might make the very idea and legitimacy of evaluation unfounded.

> In such a scenario patient satisfaction could be said to be primarily a reflection of the role patients adopt in relation to health professionals irrespective of the quality of the care itself.

Because of this dependency relationship consumers may simultaneously feel both gratitude and dissatisfaction with a service, and the quality of care may be worse than surveys of satisfaction seem to indicate. In other words, 'consumerism is dependent on a refusal to accept paternalism; it relies on the existence of consumers and not passive patients' (p 514).

The accounts given earlier in this chapter included numerous occasions when practitioners believed that clients were operating to a different agenda from the social worker. Even when they agreed with the social worker that work had gone either well or badly, the social workers sensed that client and practitioner may not have shared identical goals and may been appealing to rather different evidence. One possible explanation of this can be found in Cohen's early work with mothers with learning disabilities. Social work was viewed by some of these women as a bartering relationship, entered into for the purpose of meeting specific material needs. The relationship between the service user and the social worker was understandably regarded as part of the means to an end and not part of the end itself. He concluded,

> If social work is seen as the 'interference' one has to tolerate in order to receive the service, the consumer's evaluation may concern only a part of what the (social worker) defines as the service...We must know what the consumer sees as the boundaries of service'
>
> (Cohen, 1971: 42-43).

Our understanding of reasons why partnership in evaluating will often make heavy demands on social workers, service users and their carers has been considerably enriched by work on the sociology of neighbouring. Beginning with the seminal work of Philip Abrams, developed by other writers since his death (eg Bulmer, 1986; Bulmer

1987; Offer, 1991), attention has been drawn to the inherent tensions between formal and informal systems of care. 'Being a Good Neighbour is not the same as being a good neighbour', and in consequence the evaluation of informal care needs to draw on an understanding of the 'ideas of desert, need, responsibility, obligation and causation at the level of everyday life' (Offer, 1991: 80). Informal carers are likely to hold different views from formal carers on a large number of questions such as judgements about what counts as serious or trivial, the meaning of time scales, the adequacy or otherwise of information and advice, what counts as the most important aspect of a particular problem, how costs are evaluated, the meaning of terms in which prognoses are made, and the nature of 'progress'. Furthermore, client expectations and aspirations provide context and colour to their service evaluations, in a way which may dull criticism. Client evaluations 'are relative to context, to knowledge of services available, to expectations, to help received in past encounters, to help received from other sources, to perceptions of the "pleasantness" of the social worker' (Rees and Wallace, 1982: 72). An expression of satisfaction with a given service is a relative judgement - a comparison between aspirations and perceived status and wellbeing following social work intervention. Decontextualised measures of satisfaction are not sufficient. Social workers also need to know the nature and the service user's level of aspiration and their self-assessed personal status and wellbeing (Carr-Hill, 1992). Unless such factors are taken into account 'we can never be sure whether the high rate of client satisfaction is related more to factors like lack of knowledge or limited expectations, than the actual helpfulness of social service contact' (Rees and Wallace, 1982: 77).

The conclusion from all this is not that client and carer satisfaction judgements should be abandoned. Indeed, in Chapter Nine we outline good practice when seeking to discover client satisfaction. But satisfaction measures are not a panacea. They are difficult to interpret and utilise, and may prove politically disempowering. Narrative inquiry approaches to obtaining satisfaction overcome some of these problems by enabling social worker and service user to avoid the context-stripping tendencies of survey estimates. Social workers and participatory evaluators should resist the lure to lampoon, disparage or caricature academic studies of consumer satisfaction which are driven by a desire to add to the sum of shared human knowledge and understanding. But, just as with the advent of community care reform, service providers were increasingly expected to rethink the nature of their relationships with the people who use their services, so too social workers have to reconsider the ways in which they engage with people in evaluating their response to services. As Beresford has succinctly put it, 'there is after all rather glaring inconsistency in exploring involvement in an excluding and unparticipatory way' (Beresford, 1992: 18). Davis discovered in a comparable context that some service users described the experience of 'being researched' as similarly disempowering to their experience of being on the receiving end of insensitive services. 'Whether intrusion into your life takes place in the name of "helping" or "researching" the experience, it seems, can feel all too similar if you are on the receiving end' (Davis, 1992: 37).

Conclusion

Client and carer studies have yielded several important benefits for social work practice. We believe that such accounts - and indeed social workers' own accounts - are most helpfully viewed as narratives of experience, and neither simply 'facts' nor 'constructs'. In the majority of accounts of practice related to us, social workers did not believe that they were in harmony with clients or carers in their evaluations. Practitioners were not unduly concerned about this and often argued that such discrepancies were an irreducible quality of social work practice. In consequence, partnership in evaluating is likely to fall low on social workers' priorities, and prove difficult to achieve. We will have more to say about participatory evaluation in subsequent chapters, and we now know more about consumer satisfaction - enough to understand why satisfaction judgements are not closely related to service outcomes and client gains. The considerations we have presented provide enough ground to agree with Fisher when he concluded that

> Ratings of satisfaction cannot therefore be taken as a guide to the success of the service in meeting either its own goals or those of the clients. Such measures relate primarily to the quality of the encounter between worker and client, not to its outcome.   (Fisher, 1983: 42).

The appeal to consumer choice and satisfaction as benchmarks for evaluating the performance and quality of social work services have enjoyed a revival in connection with the reforms of community care and children's' services. In the next chapter we consider the impact of organisational and service frameworks on evaluating practice.

5 Evaluating in place

Inspectors....they're necessary;...like laxatives are necessary.

Primo Levi *('The Wrench')*

This chapter starts from the agency scene described in social workers' evaluation narratives. The scene is 'where the action occurs, where characters are formed and live out their stories and where cultural and social context play constraining and enabling roles' (Connelly and Clandinin, 1990: 8).

New and strengthened forms of managerial authority moved centre stage during the 1980s, and were intended as the vehicle through which quality would become part of the warp and woof of public sector services. We will describe practitioners' views about the characteristics and consequences of this performance culture for agency evaluation. Their judgements form both a springboard and resource bank to portray the principal features of management by effectiveness in social work, in particular, the centrality of performance measurement and the location of client outcomes at the core of organisational mission in social work. In the later pages of this chapter we will describe how practitioners viewed the relationship between their own evaluating and the work of line managers, their colleagues and other welfare professionals.

Our interest is not with debates about welfare or quality management as such (see for example Peters and Waterman, 1995; Patti, Poertner and Rapp, 1988; Connor and Black, 1994; Kirkpatrick and Lucio, 1995). Our more specific purpose is to demonstrate how cultures of management and quality constitute scenes and contexts of acute significance within which social workers construct and test evaluating in practice competencies.

Quality in the personal social services

The language of cost effectiveness, service user choice, satisfaction, empowerment, commercial models of quality management, monitoring and evaluation, service contracts and agreements, partnerships, staff supervision, financial decentralisation and assessments of outcomes permeate the present rhetoric of planning, management and delivery of British social services.

The Audit Commission report on community care in 1986 provided the benchmark for later reforms and an actuarial, value-for-money orientation to the direction of those reforms (Audit Commission, 1986). The National Health Service and Community Care Act (1990) required social services departments to produce Community Care Plans which included arrangements for quality assurance, local inspection units, complaints procedures and systems for safeguarding service standards. The Social Services Inspectorate (SSI) based in the Department of Health was given a beefed up role, and immediately began to advocate 'more explicit standards, openness, full and accurate information, choice, accountability and non-discrimination' (SSI, 1993: 3.1). There have been several themes and aspirations in the work of this national inspectorate, including the perceived need to improve the supervision of staff ('The variable quality of professional supervision is worrying'), and a shift to a managerial approach in which 'no individual fieldworker should be regarded as self sufficient' (SSI, 1992: 13).

Prominent emphasis has been placed on 'the involvement of users and carers in planning and conducting inspections, defining the criteria to be applied, and reporting the findings' (SSI, 1992: 5.4; SSI, 1995). Although satisfaction was at one point expressed by the Chief Inspector at the extent to which user involvement was taking place (SSI, 1993: 2.7), the extent to which it has been implemented is still very patchy. Only a minority of inspections have directly involved users and carers (SSI, 1994: 2.2; 3.1), and the degree to which such involvement goes beyond a consumer survey consultation and achieves some degree of advocacy and empowering is as yet very limited (SSI, 1994: 3.2).

The Home Office carried out a scrutiny of agencies and projects in the voluntary sector in 1990 which focused on performance against funding, and adopted a 'strategies expressed through objectives' approach (Home Office, 1990: 3.3). This led to the establishment of Charities Evaluation Services, intended as a nationwide resource for charity evaluation, and also stimulated voluntary agencies' interest in self-evaluation and evaluation by outsiders. Similar trends were evident in the field of supported housing and housing associations, where performance monitoring and quality assurance policies increasingly took root as the preferred tools of government funding agencies for developing and appraising supported housing. User satisfaction and tenant participation are pursued as key criteria for appraising performance in these schemes.

Following the establishment of National Standards for the supervision of offenders in the community (Home Office, 1992, 1995a), the Home Office publishes an annually revised Three Year Plan, which incorporates Key Performance Indicators against which the work of probation officers may be measured (Home Office, 1994, 1995b).

Cost-effectiveness, joint objective setting, strengthened account-ability of welfare professionals, managerial effectiveness, explicit standards, performance monitoring, and customer involvement, choice and satisfaction are recurring themes in the pleas and provisions for quality in the personal social services. These different *standards* reflect distinct underlying *approaches* to quality. Pfeffer and Coote have identified four broad approaches to quality (Pfeffer and Coote, 1991; Coote, 1994). The 'traditional' approach is based on a 'no expenses spared' concept that assesses whether one product or service is better than another. This approach is not relevant to social service provision. The second, 'scientific' approach measures quality by expert standards against which a service is assessed according to its fitness for service. The Social Services Inspectorate routinely uses a standards-based approach to evaluate services. The managerial or 'excellence' approach starts from a customer orientation as the key to service success. Rejecting mass production and mass consumption models, quality is based on demonstrating managerial effectiveness by giving the customers what they want. We have described some of the problems of this approach to consumer satisfaction in the previous chapter, but it continues to shape the government policies for a mixed economy of welfare.

Finally, the 'consumerist' approach to quality casts customers in an active role by focusing on their wishes rather than those of managers, and by seeking consumer empowerment. This approach to excellence has influenced the margins of service provision in the areas of supported housing, some voluntary agencies, a number of social services departments, and the work of some self-advocacy groups.

The meaning of quality remains elusive because it is made to serve different purposes by different people and by the same people at different times. Quality becomes a potential battle ground for both the micro- and macro-political battles of welfare provision. When the going gets tough quality as cost effectiveness is likely to appeal to funders and politicians, quality as performance control will attract managers, and the resort to quality as a mechanism for professional survival in an uncertain world will tempt practitioners. Meanings are also ambiguous because quality is often used to refer to a *process* of quality assurance, and only sometimes to a service *outcome*.

How are these developments in quality and evaluation viewed by practitioners? Evaluating in practice competencies will be exercised against the shifting backdrop of these initiatives. We have seen in Chapter Three that social workers distinguished two different kinds of evaluation - 'evaluation proper' and self-evaluation of work with service users - and that each kind of evaluation has its entirely distinctive sets of commitments, activities and attitudes. We will inspect in more detail what these social workers understood by 'evaluation proper'.

Evaluation with a capital 'E'

Evaluation proper, or 'Evaluation with a capital E' as someone else labelled it, was the term practitioners used when they wished to refer to evaluation as originating in legal or administrative requirements, planned and implemented by senior agency staff, and filtered through line managers. This model was widely regarded as being part of the change of culture we have briefly sketched, in which evaluation has become 'a big buzz word'.

> A lot of it at the end of the day, let's face it, it is just to do with the change of culture. If you've gone through, you've been working as a probation officer for ten years and you've never been asked to evaluate anything before and

> all of a sudden you are. It's like 'why? why all of a sudden?' and people get suspicious.

> Historically I think that Social Services have tended to be 'woolly' and maybe 'airy-fairy'.... Perhaps not any more, but there was a view of social workers who responded without having any clear strategy...that we were sort of bumbling and not to say incompetent...I think social workers began to wake up to that really, that we have to be more methodical and more exact in our approach.

This culture was regarded as marked by scrutiny from above, formal, occasional evaluations, a heavy time investment, quantitative measures, managerially driven expectations, and agenda stemming from general service levels rather than direct practice - 'the overall things more than the smaller bits of work' (Figure 3.1, p.38).

> The first thing you think of is somebody keeping an eye on you, somebody watching you, somebody checking on you...It's almost like testing out what skills you've got and what skills you haven't got.

> ...apprehension, that's a word I would think of. That you're being *evaluated* in terms of whether you're *performing well*, and whether you're *doing your job* well...being weighed up.

Views about 'evaluation proper'

Social workers rarely rejected this culture of evaluation out of hand. For some it was an opportunity, a way of avoiding tokenism, and a welcome added accountability.

> It is right and proper that our practice should be more rigorous and that we should have to be able to substantiate and support our judgements about people...'cos sometimes our clients are so weak and so passive and so unaware of their rights that you could traipse through their house and they wouldn't protest or wouldn't know how to.

More commonly it was accepted with resignation as an inevitable if mixed blessing.

> I genuinely welcome it. I generally get quite irritated when colleagues are resistant to the idea, in the sense that I don't think probation officers, any more than anybody else, can be immune from some sort of accountability for what we're doing. (But) I think it's perfectly possible for a probation officer to be doing very real quality work and offering a quality service, both to an individual and through that to the public, but it may not be visible in offending rates.

At worst it produced discomfort and even acute anxiety.

> Officially the current trend now is for quality and our work is going to be evaluated...Officially that has come very much to the fore...I feel very anxious about my work. It causes an anxiety to make sure my work is good, and it is going to be scrutinised.

A recurring concern was about the way official evaluations may be used to justify present inadequate resources or future cuts.

> The difficulty I think social workers are going to have is that unless they can show something tangible, in other words via evaluation, it's going to be very hard for them to have any kind of secure future...I don't know where you go, I really don't.

> I'm suspicious of it politically, about the way that statutory agencies use evaluation. I think it's a lot to do with auditing and fulfilment of targets, which really doesn't mean much when you look at the resource question. I think it's a politically inspired con.

However, the aspect of formal evaluation which led to most complaints was its perceived reliance on quantitative measures.

> The only debate that matters is, are we talking about number crunching or are we talking about quality experience?

> Evaluation in a formal way is almost more about quantity of work done than quality of work. It's a question of how many individual plans has the team got up and running rather than are they useful plans for people.

A community worker, describing performance measures for raising money for community groups, concluded,

> It does not look at how I've worked with the group, do I help them learn about how to apply for funding, do they know about codes of practice in volunteering - it doesn't actually look at that sort of evaluation. It's just a lot of figures.

The perceived impact of this culture change on quality of practice and service was viewed sceptically, for several reasons. *First*, there were doubts as to how deeply quality monitoring had permeated practice.

> I think you could probably get away for quite a long time without actually evaluating your work in any formal way. And I think your evaluation of your work would probably be believed. If you were very confident and said, 'Oh, yes, I'm really doing well on this', then I think it would be accepted.

Second, anxieties existed concerning the extent to which a deepening commitment to performance management may lead to an impoverishing of personal practice. One probation officer, while welcoming the introduction by the Home Office of National Standards as leading to greater accountability, the possibility of partnership with clients, and open file access, viewed the future with wariness.

> They're trying to get us more rigid, but not for evaluation or better practice... Evaluating your work will just be 'Yes, I've kept to National Standards. I saw them twelve times'. And that's it. You'll have done what is asked of you, but you're not evaluating good practice.

Finally, social workers believed their agencies were interested in only one *version* of evaluation, and as a consequence there were repeated instances of social workers speaking as if their personal evaluation of practice was a different animal from agency evaluation.

> The formal line, certainly coming from the Director downwards, would be that evaluation is of significance, in that the Director is always very keen on involving districts in any piece of research that may be around. It's almost a joke that if there's a piece of research going on he will want us to be involved in it.

The taken-for-granted divide between 'Evaluation with a Capital E' and practitioners' own evaluations was expressed in a probation officer's enthusiastic account of the benefits gained by members of a group for offenders. She added several times 'they have been evaluated separately within the organisation, but I haven't seen the results of that.' She thought 'anecdotally' that the reoffending rate for the group members was very low, but had neither followed up the story or apparently been given the feedback from the programme evaluators. Social workers had little familiarity with the identifiable outcomes of their work - 'I'm still working in the dark'. The agency apparatus of monitoring and performance measures did not support or enable evaluating in practice. As one community worker succinctly put it, 'I don't think it's difficult. I think it hasn't been done. It hasn't been policy.'

These practitioners were reflecting on their awareness of important changes in management objectives and style. What are the main features of these changes, and what impact are they likely to have on social workers' evaluating practice?

Management by effectiveness

Advocacy of quality management within the personal social services has led to an emphasis on accountability, rigour, and a demand for thought out evidencing of professional claims. This much was clear from almost all the social workers to whom we spoke. It is also apparent from experience reported from elsewhere. Citizens' anxieties about standards of service have been drawn into the public arena, and channels provided for earlier disclosure of unacceptable practices. Quality management has stimulated some instances of good practice involving practitioners, managers and service users (James, Brooks and Towell, 1992). For example, the ENQUIRE System of quality assurance developed by the King's Fund includes the establishment of Quality Action Groups, where professionals, users, carers, volunteers and others work together to evaluate the impact of different services, and where the information is presented in a way which is more likely to facilitate participation by users (Richards and Heginbotham, 1992).

User involvement also has been prominent in the work of the Birmingham Community Care Special Action project, the results of which have been widely disseminated through the publications of the Leeds based Nuffield Institute for Health Services Studies. The work of Croft and Beresford has added to the awareness of the potential of participatory evaluation methods, and citizen-involvement research (Beresford, 1992; Beresford and Croft, 1993).

Evaluating in practice work by social workers will be informed and enriched by these developments. However, the responses of the social workers to whom we spoke make clear that there are certain characteristics of the performance culture which may not prove uniformly positive for service users or practitioners. Social workers and service users need to draw their own conclusions about ways in which practice evaluation is shaped by government, the possibilities for negative consequences of a commitment to managing by measurement, and the potential within quality management for the emergence of tokenistic as well as genuinely empowering forms of user involvement.

Government and evaluation

There is a tradition of applied government social research in Britain stretching back to the Royal Commission on the Poor Laws in 1832, continuing with major programmes of poverty research later in the last century, and extending through research on education early in the present century. An informed American commentator has observed how the characteristic British tendency to nurture secrecy in their operations has effected evaluation. The 1980s witnessed a shift of control of research from the universities to central government. Consequently government departments 'considered studies to be departmental property, conducted for the departments rather than for the general interest' (House, 1993: 43).

Under the Thatcher governments professional autonomy became subsumed under managerial authority. Within western governments evaluation programmes provide one means of legitimating authority by providing guidance and achieving compliance. In return government provides legitimisation for evaluation, which becomes an increasingly valuable commodity in a period when evaluation is becoming increasingly professionalised. Active Evaluation Societies now exist in America, Canada, Australia, Britain and Europe, and postgraduate level training in evaluation is emerging in British universities. Social workers' personal evaluating in practice skills will be developed in a political context where it can be argued that the promotion of partnership arrangements between public and voluntary sector agencies marks a major and worrying shift in relations between the state and the voluntary sector (Shaw, 1995), and in organisational contexts where planned evaluation is likely to occupy an increasingly institutionalised role.

Managing by measurement

It is not simply a growth in managerial authority that has taken place, but the development of a particular kind of managerialism. The perceived preoccupation of 'evaluation proper' with quantity rather than quality and worth was perhaps the single most frequently expressed anxiety among the social workers whose narratives have provided the spine for the first part of this book. Social workers

> resent applying quantitative systems of measurement to their work and have often responded angrily that number counts do not easily really tell the story of what they do...Practitioners resent these systems because they do not take into account the difficulty of the case or the level of skill required to achieve desired outcomes.
>
> (Grasso and Epstein, 1988: 93).

This resentment is given short shrift by enthusiasts of the management by effectiveness school. Walter Hudson drew the uncompromising conclusions that 'if you cannot measure a client's problem, it does not exist...if you cannot measure a client's problem, you cannot treat it...if you cannot measure an intervention, it does not exist...if you cannot measure an intervention, you cannot administer it' (Hudson, 1988). Effectiveness managers reject as myths the views that human service outcomes are idiosyncratic, that outcomes cannot readily be measured, that practitioners cannot be held accountable for client outcomes, or that outcome evaluation takes too much in the way of time and resources (Rapp and Poertner, 1988).

The quotation from Hudson is, of course, not directly about management but about social work practice. A knot of logically similar social work methods, management approaches, and evaluation strategies clusters around management by effectiveness. An example of this can be observed in the British Probation Service. A series of conferences was held for Probation managers, Home Office officials, probation officers and academics under the theme 'What Works?'. Major papers from the conferences have been published (McGuire, 1995). The intertwining themes within these conferences were a resurgent confidence that quasi-experimental research methods can demonstrate the effectiveness of intervention; that behavioural and cognitive approaches, with their emphasis on structure, goals, operationalised skills, and empirically based practice, offer a route to demonstrable effectiveness; and a belief that management by measurement finds a direct analogue in quasi-experimental research methods. Management is believed to mirror research and research to mirror practice.

There are several important strengths of this approach. Rapp and Poertner's complaint that 'agency and programme goals are almost always stated in terms of what will the agency do or provide rather than on the specific benefits to be accrued by clients as a result of these agency efforts' is not unreasonable. Managers who are 'single-minded, and obsessed with clients' (1988: 24) are preferable to agency information systems dominated by amounts of service provided, numbers and types of clients served and so forth. But is a management by measurement strategy likely to achieve these goals? There are a number of considerations that pose unresolved doubts, and which in particular raise the question whether strict management by effectiveness approaches create a self defeating threat to the development of practitioners' evaluating in practice competencies.

- managing by measurement risks producing a concentration on easily measurable aspects of practice.

- organisational behaviour will change in order to score well on measurable criteria.

- agency performance requirements will take precedence at the expense of the service user.

- the professional role of the social worker is put at jeopardy by management through measurement.

- conflicts are created within line manager, middle manager and senior manager roles.

- the argument that good *management* practice and good *evaluation* practice are logically closely similar is oversimple.

Etzioni remarked long ago that 'frequent measuring tends to encourage over-production of measurable items and neglect of less measurable items' (Etzioni, 1964: 9). Conrad, describing the extensive annual Programme Assessment System which New York's foster care agencies were required to operate, wryly noted how performance statistics resulted in precisely this negative, unintended consequence (Conrad, 1985). Plans, contracts, placements, numbers of visits, and other more easily measured outputs gained higher profiles within social work agencies, and informal or less easily measured aspects of practice became invisible. A similar example can be seen ten years on from Conrad's study, in that only one of the Home Office Key Performance Indicators for probation officers requires a qualitative measure.

It is an easy but significant step from this to a position where the organisation changes its behaviour in order to score well on those criteria. Numbers become reified as true indicators of quality. The organisation will seek to control intakes and jettison 'weak' cases, and agency members will be tempted to distort how the work of the agency appears.

Conrad's salutary vignette illustrates how accountability systems can serve to undermine the quality of care they were mandated and developed to protect and enhance - 'the very individuals the reforms aim to rescue can become the victims of its remedy' (Conrad, 1985: 642). Decision makers were tempted to place the agency's performance requirements above the best interests of the child. For example, in order to achieve programme targets, children were sometimes reunited with families when professional judgement would suggest the contrary. Specialist agencies were known on occasion to refuse to accept deeply troubled children as a means of avoiding the risk of performing poorly. Thus, while accountability standards of the kind increasingly generated in British social work are doubtless partly intended to codify good practice, these requirements may 'encourage agency personnel to make decisions for which the agency will be rewarded, good casework practice or not, and to avoid those for which sanctions will result' (p646). It is hard, therefore, to dissent from Grasso and Epstein's conclusion that 'emphasis on quantitative measures of effectiveness and efficiency has resulted in a number of different types of goal distortion and displacement' (1988: 89).

In the longer term, management by measurement is likely to exercise a negative influence on the role of social workers. The pressure to over-conformity, excessive caution and even falsification of information, removes the freedom to doubt and, in the words of one English director of social services, will be experienced as a 'checklists and truncheons' approach. William Reid has suggested that if social workers focus their energy on the achievement of effective but probably modest results, this can 'discourage more radical but possibly less testable innovations'. He goes on to ask, 'Is it better to make limited but well documented progress or to work toward more important goals with less certainty of what we have attained?' (Reid, 1988: 45). Reid's conclusion, drawing on long experience of developing and evaluating task centred practice models, is based on a belief that evaluation, quality measurement and management are not, after all, easy bedfellows. The social workers to whom we spoke were right in their belief that evidence in social work often is not easy to interpret, and cannot be incorporated into management prescriptions in an uncomplicated way. In Reid's chastening if memorable metaphor,

> It is like trying to decide which horse won a close race viewed at a bad angle from the grandstand during a cloudburst

(Reid, 1988: 48).

In this light, the words of a senior probation manager at a What Works? conference, albeit spoken from the floor, sound slightly chilling. Speaking of probation officers, this manager said, 'someone out there is cancelling out the good effects. It makes me angry.

Whoever is producing those bad results has to be stopped'. The comment points up the neglect of ethical considerations which marks management by effectiveness models. We are not, of course, suggesting that managers committed to effectiveness approaches are less ethical than managers and practitioners of other schools, but rather are marking the refusal of consistent proponents of effectiveness models to recognise that managerial choices directed by ethical considerations may detract from as well as enhance service effectiveness. A manager who is 'devoid of guile, free of cant, not given to manipulative relationships' (Lewis, 1988), may, Lewis reasonably points out, decide to limit workloads in order to lessen burdens on highly stressed staff, and so reduce the number of clients that can be served. She may also decide to give preferential treatment to a worker not on the basis of merit but on the basis of the needs of the organisation. Thus adherence to ethical principles *may* prove detrimental to service effectiveness.

> It is entirely possible that a manager who acts in an ethically commendable fashion may contribute to a less effective service for some and a more effective service for others
>
> (Lewis, 1988: 282).

We should not overstate the scale of these changes. Evidence suggests, perhaps not surprisingly, that the rhetoric of management is honoured as often in the breach as in the observance (Shaw, 1995). The possibility of superficial implementation is probably what was referred to when someone aptly described this management style within the Probation Service as being 'pretty on the ball' (Humphrey and Pease, 1992: 48). However, real changes have taken place in the role of managers within the personal social services, and quality management has some way to go before it burns out.

Client centred management

We noted in the previous chapter that the organisational restructuring of social work in England and Wales in the late 1980's included a recasting of users and carers as participants with a role to play in defining what questions should be asked. However, 'concepts of user-oriented and user-led services are more strongly to be observed in rhetoric than practice' (Barnes and Wistow, 1992: 8). The conclusion drawn from an early review of quality assurance practices in social services departments was that,

Again and again we found definitions of quality assurance in use and evidence of standard setting which overwhelmingly represented the views of managers and professionals rather than those of service users

(James, Brooks and Towell, 1992: 2.1).

Choice for service users is limited by lack of geographical mobility, inability to choose any different option because many are involuntary clients, and by the existence of service monopolies especially in the case of specialist services. Providers also need to be sensitive to the demands they place on users whose lives are already complex and demanding. Barnes and Wistow quote a woman who wrote when returning an evaluation questionnaire to the Birmingham Special Action project, 'because of the situation I am in, sometimes it is hard to find *time* or *mind* to sit and fill in forms or write letters. After caring for someone all you want to do is rest' (Barnes and Wistow, 1992: 99).

Unless a heavily cynical view is adopted, this potential marginalisation of the user is not what was intended by the framers of the Children Act, 1989 and the community care reforms. 'Both aim to replace systems dominated by professionals with approaches based on partnership with service users...The focus...has been on ways of making it easier for children, parents, users and carers to participate and be heard' (SSI, 1992: 5.2,3). '*Caring for People*', however embryonically, did provide an opportunity for working towards genuine user partnership, representation and accountability.

User involvement does, of course, cover a range of possible meanings, best viewed as lying on a continuum from self-advocacy to consumerist models (Beresford, 1992). Self-advocacy approaches have a clear commitment to promoting the empowerment of users, and extending their capacity to participate in decisions about the design, management and review of services. Consumerist strategies tend to be more service provider led and are targeted at improving the quality of services by making them more responsive and sensitive.

User involvement strategies are also clarified by disaggregating the broad category of 'user'. Even if users are distinguished from carers, there remain important distinctions between voluntary and involuntary users, long and short-term users, and current and potential users (Barnes and Wistow, 1992). Client groups may be in competition with each other, and users are also citizens. 'We are interested as citizens in planning and as customers in delivery' (Pfeffer and Coote, 1991: 26). The distinction between voluntary and involuntary service users is given too little recognition in the language of consumerism. Fisher refers to two kinds of problem that occur, and which mean that 'allegiance to agreements is not matched by practice particularly when the user is involuntary or at risk' (Fisher, 1992: 58). The problem of what Fisher calls the *'third mandate'* occurs where explicit legal sanction for action is missing, but intervention is imposed on the client, as when case conferences or reviews take place. The problem of *escalation* occurs when the original mandate gets extended to other areas. Agreements with involuntary clients tend to be coercive, conditional or constrained by resource problems. Passive consent is too often taken to mean agreement. Fisher wisely warns that 'we must avoid interpreting consent to an offer of a single resource or service as a positive choice' and 'resist the temptation to use 'word-magic' to rewrite user compliance as positive choice' (p60, 61).

Our interest in the growth of user involvement lies, as we have suggested, in the consequences of such developments for social workers' evaluating in practice. User involvement that is to any degree committed to empowerment will include the development of quality and performance measures based on criteria defined by users and carers, and user participation in the evaluation process. 'A more participatory agency practice begs a more participatory research' (Beresford, 1992: 18). Feedback by and to users and carers, described by Weissman as 'one of the most profound changes that can be introduced into a social agency' (Weissman, 1988: 218), will emerge as an inevitable ingredient of user involvement in evaluation.

Supervisors, colleagues and other professionals

We have unpacked the shifts in relations between social work and the state, the development of tighter management styles, the potential for user participation, and the significance of these developments for the agency scenes and contexts in which social workers will develop evaluating in practice competencies. Each of these themes is connected with motifs in social workers' narratives of evaluation. These social workers practised across a very wide range of agencies, organisations and projects. Yet they were at one in carrying round an image of 'evaluation proper' - a formal, planned, largely quantitative, performance-related, activity carried out from above by 'strangers' to satisfy larger agency agenda. While this is not the only model of evaluating held by social workers, it becomes of central significance when we consider the characters that people the social context occupied by social workers - the impact of colleagues, team members, line managers, and social workers in other agencies on evaluating in practice.

Supervision - evaluating or caretaking?

Do social workers discuss their work during supervision sessions or formal team meetings from the standpoint of evaluation? If not, does supervision have the potential for such discussion? If evaluating *is* part of supervision, do practitioners think their line managers share their own view about the work they have done?

The only occasion that evaluation was mentioned in the context of regular team meetings was when one child protection social worker said that statistics about children were

> presented to us on a monthly basis at a team meeting, but it's usually quite perfunctory really. It's sort of, well, you know, 'We've just had these figures and we're down this month or we're up', you know. 'You can have a look at them if you like. They're in my drawer.'

Social workers were not always confident that they knew how line managers viewed their practice. 'I think the manager understood my position, but maybe he would have approached it from a totally different angle', was a typical response. Those who received supervision were unanimous - 'there's very little emphasis on evaluation in supervision.' Evaluation was not discussed in supervision, except perhaps in some informal, tacit sense. The system often militated against supervision being used to that end, but some social workers believed good grounds existed for strengthening the evaluative dimension of supervision. What evidence did they cite to support the different elements of this argument?

Two child protection social workers said that supervision, 'can tend to be just a gallop through the cases, with occasional looks at personal development.' Evaluation is never raised 'as a separate issue'. 'I think my supervisor relies on me and other social workers to evaluate our own practice, and relies on us to say to her, "You have to close this case now".' This style of supervision was labelled 'caretaking' by one community worker, and several social workers felt that the system militated against the possibility of critical evaluation within supervision.

> I don't know that she has really *evaluated* my role in this... I mean, she's been quite supportive. But I'm not really convinced that she's interested in giving me a negative evaluation of my work at the moment. So I think she's gonna look for the positive. Whereas I think I'm more concerned about the outcome for the client and the family, and that I could have done more to help.

A probation officer advanced a similar argument.

> I think supervision sessions have a tendency to be quite collusive. There's an overview - 'Are you managing your workload? Are the reports being done on time?', and that kind of thing. That seems to be the general gist of supervision, not 'Let's look at these pieces of work' and 'How good were they? Were they effective? Did you achieve...?', you know those kind of things.

The inference that supervision is somehow failing by its neglect of evaluating was reinforced by the occasional advocacy of a shift towards more formal evaluation. But there was a belief, in the words of one child protection social worker, that 'in practical reality, if you get through your cases and look at the plans you're making, that's probably as much as you're gonna get.' This is consistent with our knowledge that social workers are more likely than line managers to criticise the adequacy of supervision (eg Payne, 1994). The important point here, however, is not whether the supervision was genuinely good or bad, but the degree to which evaluation was not seen to be a part of the process.

Evaluating with colleagues

If supervision gave fairly minimal emphasis to evaluation, collegial evaluation was almost non-existent.

> We don't do it. I'm being honest with you because I feel that the material you get will get people to change their attitudes...There's a lot of mystique around social work, and I suppose it's like any profession in that you guard the information that you have.

The only exception to this was occasional localised utilisation of a mutual gatekeeping process in the Probation Service to appraise pre-sentence reports before they were presented. At its most effective this process has substantial advantages. It enables a close monitoring of anti-discriminatory practice in report writing, promotes a close and mutually satisfying collaboration between practitioners and managers, and takes forward a practical collaborative ethos.

> We gatekeep on all reports on first offenders, female offenders and black offenders, because we feel they're the most discriminated against in the court system...We feel it should be part of every report.

Another probation officer was more sceptical about gatekeeping. 'You're asking people with an emotional relationship to evaluate each other.' However, several social workers went out of their way to advocate the development of such approaches.

> It would be much more valuable if we shared some of it more closely between us all, which we don't tend to do. We don't get together and maybe say 'This is a difficult case for me, let's talk about it for half an hour'.

> Sometimes it would be useful to have other people to tease out what it is about today that makes you feel bad about that piece of work you've done.

A community worker described enthusiastically the only reported description of such peer evaluation.

> Working with him helps me look at what I'm doing. What I'll do is I'll help him evaluate me. I'll come in and say, 'Oh, that was terrible', and he'll say, 'Well, what happened?'. I'll tell him and he'll say, 'Mmh no, it wasn't that bad. Well have you thought of this?,' and I'll do the same for him. It's really good we share because he's so different to me, so we sort of complement each other.

How others do it

Widespread uncertainty existed among the social workers we spoke to regarding the practice and agenda of evaluation outside the field with which the social worker was directly familiar. As far as their knowledge extended, they were of the view that the basic issues about evaluation were fairly similar from one social work agency to another. There were frequent comments to the effect that evaluation was probably more or less explicit, tight or precise in other settings, but the underlying tenor of social workers' views was that 'we've all got slightly different corners but all come together at the centre.'

This consensus sometimes carried over to include other professions apart from social work. More commonly, however, the view was that social workers had a relatively tough job when it came to evaluating. Health visitors could weigh a baby, paediatricians could log when a child started to speak, but social workers had the job of measuring intangibles such as coping.

Common ground did not preclude the possibility of sharp differences over evaluating any given problem, and several social workers referred to the dilemmas that can occur in situations when participants have their own beliefs about who should be the beneficiary of intervention. 'Everyone's got different objectives', and practitioners recognise the risk of "getting sucked into their stuff".'

> The criteria do vary depending on who you're working with and where their interests actually lie within a piece of work.

This often occurred in child protection cases where the conflict was between the needs of the child and those of the mother. 'It doesn't always have to be a positive end with the family for me to feel that I've done a good piece of work - it's whether the child's protected.'

Conclusion

A changed and strengthened management style was intended by Conservative governments to provide the vehicle through which quality management was made part of the warp and woof of the personal social services. Managers in social work have traditionally been in a powerful position relative to practitioners (Howe, 1991), and the introduction of management by effectiveness poses the risk that social work management will be moulded into a rational straightjacket. Most social workers probably came to accept, as part of their training, a critique of professional power - a critique of excessive claims and limited achievements, failures of professional responsibility, absence of professional neutrality, trampling on citizens' rights, lack of accountability and so on (Wilding, 1982). In a policy climate where governments have answered 'precisely so' to this battery of criticism, this presents an opening for a potentially damaging transformation of professional roles in social work. While it may be too early to reach a firm judgement (Kirkpatrick and Martinez, 1995), Pfeffer and Coote were in no doubt that 'one of the main effects of the changes has been to begin to limit the power of the 'caring' professionals' (Pfeffer and Coote, 1991: 12) . Pitts vociferously complained to similar effect that some applications of the justice model within the field of supervision of offenders in the community have resulted in probation becoming deprofessionalised. Probation officers, he suggests, have voluntarily become technicians and risk entering a 'state of voluntary conceptual amnesia' (Pitts, 1992: 146).

The quality of relations between social workers and first line managers - 'the buffer between accountability on the one hand and client demands on the other' (Grasso and Epstein, 1988: 94) - is one key measure of social workers' chances of developing the critical culture necessary if evaluating in practice competencies are to flourish, and they are to avoid the risk of becoming technicians, against which Pitts and others have warned. Yet social workers whose accounts are found in the previous paragraphs were uncertain of what they hoped for from supervision, and had little clear idea how their own first line managers viewed the evaluation role within supervision.

These social workers were doubtless reflecting a wider uncertainty within social work regarding the purpose, function and quality of supervision. Line managers are commonly expected to carry our both a supervising role and a consultancy role (Payne, 1994). Supervision involves monitoring daily functioning, administrative management, and periodic appraisals of practice. Consultation entails staff development together with a support role. Inclusion of practitioners' evaluating in practice within supervision probably falls on a sensitive border between supervision and consultation. Supervisors do not enjoy a management role, and some of the best evidence about the process of supervision suggests that good work is demonstrated through an interactive process of 'telling the case' and not simply by matching the performance of staff against agency objectives (Pithouse, 1987). Supervision is in many instances probably 'infrequent, rushed and separated from management responsibilities' (Payne, 1994: 54). Practice teachers have been required since the early 1990's to obtain direct, first-hand evidence about students' performance. Direct evidence of this kind is very uncommon in social work staff supervision.

In this context of frequent superficiality and ambiguity of purpose, it is not at all clear that exhortations to 'do better' and change supervision practices would have any immediate impact. The methods of evaluating in practice that we outline in the second part of this book suggest that the development of these professional competencies is more likely to take place through exchange with colleagues and service users.

Management by effectiveness models, while they represent a strong commitment to client benefits, are characterised by serious weaknesses. They do not give due recognition to the difficulties of gaining evidence about social work practice and suppose a misleading analogy between social work practice, management, and evaluation. They are also insufficiently sensitive to the goal displacement that results from tight accountability systems, have a potentially withering effect on professional roles in welfare, and give inadequate weight to ethical considerations in management and social work practice. Evaluating in practice competencies overlaps at several points with the customer orientation found in management by effectiveness strategies, but we will outline in the following chapter how they are based on a set of commitments that follows a parallel course at some points but diverges at many others.

6   Valuing evaluation

It's making me have to think very **hard**. You know. About things that you just don't think about on a day-to-day basis.

Well, no, I **do** think. Obviously I think about these things. It's not that I don't think about these things, but, to have to pin myself down...I suppose it really shows up how little I think about my work on a serious, profound level.

Probation officer

White coat and purple coat
a sleeve from both he sews.
That white is always stained with blood,
that purple by the rose.

A phantom rose and blood most real
compose a hybrid style;
white coat and purple coat
few men can reconcile.

White coat and purple coat
can each be worn in turn
but in the white a man will freeze
and in the purple burn.

Dannie Abse ('Song for Pythagoras')

Evaluating in practice has received almost no attention in the teaching, delivery and management of social work practice. There are occasional exceptions, the most prominent being the emergence of the empirical practice movement in America, and the associated advocacy of single system practice evaluation. Social workers make a choice between versions of rigour or relevance. Most opt for 'the swampy lowlands of experience, trial and error, intuition and muddle through'. A small minority opt for the 'high, hard ground' of precise and narrowly technical practice (Schon, 1983).

The sketch of the main defining features of evaluating in practice strategies which opens this chapter raises several key questions which lie near the heart of much contemporary debate about the purpose of social work, in particular how can practitioners demonstrate commitment to both understanding and action. Shunning most of the 'high, hard ground', we will argue that the answers to these questions lies in the development of reflexive practice, plausible evidence, evaluating for and with the service user, anti-discriminatory evaluating, and evaluative purposefulness. These qualities of practice will provide a sequence of 'floating stepping stones' (Altheide and Johnson, 1994: 490) around the swampy lowlands, that enable us to explore rather different versions of both rigour and relevance. Our procedure offers an exploratory basis on which a plausible and adequate account of evaluating in practice can be accomplished. Practice expressions of evaluating in practice sketched out in the next three chapters - sketched as 'cartoons', outline animations and no more - indicate the kind of evaluating skills that seem to follow from the more general discussion in this chapter.

Evaluating in practice

Evaluating in practice is both evaluating *on* practice and evaluating-in-practice. As evaluating on practice it is practice recollected or anticipated in relative tranquillity. As evaluating-in-practice it rejects 'clinical impressionism' and entails the 'disciplined subjectivity' (Erikson, 1959) partly captured by one of our respondents who spoke of thinking on your feet, and by the accounts that social workers gave us of working to a 'game plan', 'knowing your prey', and good timing.

Evaluating in practice is a social rather than a solitary activity. Social in the commonsense meaning that social work is a collective activity, with negotiated purposes and consequences, but social also in several other equally important senses. As to its *purpose* it is, as we explore later, evaluation *for* others. As to its characteristic *process*, it is evaluation *with* others. Evaluating in practice has important private as well as public dimensions, and this includes collective work with community groups (Henderson and Thomas, 1980*)*. Yet it is no less a social action for being private. We might have described this as 'interpretive' or 'critical' evaluation if these labels did not tend to a kind of sloganising that causes us acute discomfort, and which gives a number of hostages to fortune.

The evaluating practitioners' knowing is *in* their action. In an important passage, Donald Schon (1983: 50) summarises part of what this means for good professional practice.

> In his day-to-day practice he makes innumerable judgements of quality for which he cannot state adequate criteria, and he displays skills for which he cannot state the rules and procedures. Even when he makes conscious use of research-based theories and techniques, he is dependent on tacit assumptions, judgements and skilful performances.
>
> On the other hand, both ordinary people and professional practitioners often think about what they are doing, sometimes even while doing it. Stimulated by surprise, they turn thought back on action and on the knowing which is implicit in the action...As (the professional) tries to make sense of it, he also reflects on the understandings which have been implicit in his action, understandings which he surfaces, restructures and embodies in further action.
>
> It is this entire process of reflection-in-action which is central to the 'art' by which practitioners deal well with situations of uncertainty, instability, uniqueness and value conflict.

There are weaknesses in this way of understanding evaluating in practice. First, Schon does not sufficiently recognise that evaluating in practice possesses an essential collaborative dimension. It is done *with* as well as for people. Second, there is a gender-blindness running through his argument in which hierarchical relationships are always rendered as he-to-she, and which never inspects gender as a dimension of evaluating. Third, he tends to treat all decisions as if they were novel and unique. This fails to acknowledge that some decisions are routine rather than novel. This becomes important when we consider evaluating assessment and planning in the next chapter. 'Routine' does not equal decisions made without any thinking. Bloor makes clear from his analysis of decisions made by adeno-tonsillectomy consultants that routine clinical decisions require both decision rules and procedures for searching information. Neither are routine decisions simple ones. Finally, we should not assume that practitioners will always agree about routine decisions. Bloor's work revealed major differences between consultants and he concludes that routines are in large part 'specialist-specific' (Bloor, 1978).

Yet despite these significant reservations Schon's statement of reflection-in-action is an important one and captures the following qualities of evaluating in practice,

- it is a disciplined activity in which the sources of understanding and action are not automatically picked off the surface, but which are *tacit*. Skilful action 'often reveals 'a knowing more than we can say" (p51).

- evaluating in practice involves a *reflexivity* - 'a bending back on itself' - and a *testing* by reflection. Erikson's injunction is entirely apt. We should be constantly trying to 'force favourite assumptions to become probable inferences' (1959: 94).

- there is an inherent comparability between 'professional' and 'ordinary', lay persons' capacities for displaying the ingredients of evaluating in practice. Professional competencies are not hermetically sealed, special abilities.

He also invites comparison between evaluating in social work and evaluating in other professions. Schon is not advancing a case simply about social work but about 'a fundamental structure of professional inquiry' (p130) encompassing social workers and architects, planners and teachers. That comparison lies outside the scope of this book, but points to helpful avenues of possible understanding and action.

Schon's starting point is knowing in action. Good evaluatings in practice reveal *tacit knowledge* - 'the largely unarticulated, contextual understanding that is often manifested in nods, silences, humour and naughty nuances' (Altheide and Johnson, 1994: 492). There are actions, judgements and recognitions which we know how to carry out spontaneously. We do not have to think about them prior to performance. We are often unaware of having learned to do them. While we may remember once being aware of the understanding necessary for action, we typically are now unable to describe the knowing which our actions reveal. In the empirical work that tracks through the first part of this book we were inviting people to reflect *on* their knowing-in-practice, to surface and review their largely tacit, 'thinking as usual' knowledge (the phrase is Alfred Schutz's, 1971). Altheide and Johnson are writing about good *ethnographies*, but their words (p492) will translate and 'stand for' this basic ingredient of evaluating in practice, just as they would for the heightened awareness between lovers.

> Tacit knowledge exists in that time when action is taken that is not understood, when understanding is offered without articulation, and when conclusions are apprehended without an argument.

One implication of this is that written accounts and texts of evaluating in practice do not provide an exhaustive statement of what such evaluating means, because written text often overlooks the subtle and significant role of tacit knowledge. The problem for this largely non-discursive knowledge is 'how to talk about what is seldom spoken about' (Altheide and Johnson, 1994: 493).

Schon unpacks reflection-in-action in terms of answers to four questions. First, how do social workers 'set' problems and evaluate their problem setting? Second, how do practitioners bring past experience to bear on a unique situation? Third, how should good evaluating in practice exhibit rigour? Finally, what is entailed in a critical stance towards inquiry?

Hugh England, in his valuable discussion of 'Social Work as Art', analyses what constitutes a rounded description and appraisal of practice, and in doing so provides a stimulating comment on the first of these four questions. He perhaps goes too far when he concludes that 'without adequate description there can be no possibility of evaluation' (England, 1986: 155), but his assertion is helpful for good practice because without such description we certainly will not force our favourite assumptions to become probably inferences. He rightly insists that social work practice 'must be subject to a description and analysis which can determine quality' (p139). It has to be described in such a way that it renders access to and evaluation of its strengths and weaknesses feasible. By making clear the links between 'understanding, action and effect' (p154), practitioners will be able to conclude whether they have 'plausibly and adequately' helped.

For instance, whether or not they are able to reach agreement, social workers, service users, carers, colleagues, first line managers and others who are part of the change agent system, need to make explicit the 'inventories of evidential signs they regularly but unwittingly scan' (Erikson, 1959: 82) if understanding is to lead to change, and change lead to understanding.

Inadequate work, England suggests, will fail to make clear the links between understanding and effect. It may identify objectives and outcomes, but offer no scope for linking the two. Even on occasions where service users' wellbeing improves, it will not be shown to be ultimately rooted in the worker's practice. He describes an example of 'sufficiently successful social work' which he concludes made possible an evaluation of the worker's practice because it

> offers access which permits evaluation of both understanding and action; it is possible from this account to assent to or dissent from the worker's stance because so much relevant information is given (p198).

If our practice cannot be challenged, we have not evaluated in practice.

Schon proposes that new 'cases' are unique entities made up of familiar categories. So, in answering his *second* question about bringing past experience to bear, he suggests that practitioners build up a repertoire of examples, images, understandings and actions. For social workers these will include accounts and stories of problems, attempted solutions and so on. In making sense of a new situation the practitioner '*sees* it *as* something already present in his repertoire.' The unfamiliar is seen 'as both similar to and different from the familiar...The familiar situation functions as a precedent, or...an exemplar of the unfamiliar one' (Schon, 1985: 138).

Schon answers his *third* question about rigour in evaluating by claiming that good practice operates as different forms of experiment, ranging from 'the probing, playful activity by which we get a feel for things' (p145) to a kind of hypothesis testing that proceeds by acting as if something were true. 'The inquirer's relation to this situation is *transactional*. He shapes the situation, but in conversation with it, so that his own models and appreciations are also shaped by the situation...He is *in* the situation that he seeks to understand' (p150-151).

What is entailed in a critical stance towards enquiry? Our own answer to this *fourth* question lies in terms of seeing evaluating in practice as a series of commitments. In brief, it involves making ourselves and our evaluating in practice accountable, and, as suggested in the introductory chapter, keeping social work honest. Our evaluatings will never exhaust the meaning of the situation, which will have a life of its own distinct from our intentions, and which may foil our projects and reveal new meanings. We do not simply shape the situation. We need constantly to keep a 'double-vision' and hold ourselves open to the situation's 'talk-back' (Schon, 1985: 163, 164). Fail in this and evaluating in practice is no longer a genuine practice competence because it cannot be understanding for action, it will preclude evaluating with others, and it will render impossible the practice goal that 'the process of the evaluation becomes an outcome in its own right' (Barnes and Wistow, 1992: 13).

This account of evaluating in practice raises at least as many questions as it answers - questions of what is meant by a reflexive practice, whether evaluating with and for service users must be in some senses a partisan and committed activity, how do we judge whether evaluations are plausible and adequate, what is required for anti-discriminatory evaluating in practice? But before we tackle these questions, there is an issue which we have so far implicitly bracketed. Probably all of the writers we have cited so far in this chapter would contrast their own approaches with a different approach which they would describe as positivism. Schon, for instance, explicitly dis- sociates his argument from the 'technical rationality' which he describes as 'the heritage of positivism' (p31). But does good evaluating in practice - indeed good social work - require a rejection of positivism?

Parenthesis: positivism - slaying the dragon

Positivism is dead. It's death is not mourned. Any continuing move- ment is akin to that of a headless chicken. Social workers have often read the announcement in the deaths column of practice texts. Indeed, the frequency and character of references to positivism in social work literature are remarkable, though they are almost always directed at others. The references to positivism in social work are almost always negative and often angry, as when the broadside is fired that 'positivists not only see their work as uncontaminated: they see themselves as pure and safe in their objectivity, an elite who have managed to transcend the constraints of subjectivity' (Everitt, Hardiker, Littlewood and Mullender, 1992:6). 'We reject positivism as a theory of knowledge and a methodology for getting to know' might have been spoken on behalf of the majority of social workers in the West (p23). It is 'a swearword by which no-one is swearing' (Williams, 1976). Among the few who are willing to swear, Bruce Thyer has argued that social work based on positivism provides a means by which effective practice can be achieved, and seen to be achieved.

> Our clients deserve the best services our profession can provide, and for the determination of social work effectiveness there is no substitute for controlled experimental research, guided by the philosophy of science known as logical positivism and the tenets of the hypothetico-deductive process
>
> (Thyer, 1989: 320).

Thyer's proposition suggest the principles upon which positivism is based, which include,

1.   The *scientific method*. Positivists claim that the methods of the natural sciences are applicable to the social sciences. The fact that the subjects of such research are human is said to make no difference to the logic of investigation.

2.   *Empiricism* expressed in an emphasis on method in science. Reality consists in what is available to the senses, and ideas are tested against what is observable. Claims to knowledge that go beyond this are rejected as meaningless.

3.   *Objectivism*. A strong distinction is drawn between facts and values. Science can only produce factual knowledge, and can neither evaluate nor prescribe. Sheldon expresses this position clearly in suggesting that 'our thinking about the concepts of effectiveness becomes muddled when we try to deal with technical questions of validity and reliability alongside moral questions' (Sheldon, 1986: 225). This objectivism usually carries with it an aversion to metaphysics, and sometimes a programme of extending scientific knowledge to society. Practice knowledge is not a different kind of knowledge such as craft or art, but applied scientific knowledge.

Positivism has been undermined from inside and out, and the arguments are a familiar part of the literature (eg Heineman, 1981). Yet the propensity of some social work writers to use 'positivism', along with its companions 'empiricism', 'scientism' and 'objectivism', as global swearwords and slogans is unhelpful. In this connection Hammersley has criticised the tendency to talk of positivism as a 'paradigm', because it implies that all the characteristics of positivism come as a package, and also that there are no internal differences.

'It obscures both potential and actual diversity in orientation, and can lead us into making simplistic methodological decisions' (Hammersley, 1995: 3). For example, the authors of a contemporary text which helpfully seeks to promote research-minded social work practice, claim that one of the problems of 'the positivist paradigm' is that 'the research endeavour is mystified; esoteric skills and techniques serve the interests of the powerful.' They reach the conclusion that 'the essential values of positivism, objectivity, neutrality and determinism are...at variance with the value base, and the purposeful and humble activities of social work practice' (Everitt, Hardiker, Littlewood and Mullender, 1992: 35, 55, 61), and that those whose research is framed by positivism are guilty of 'spurious and dangerously simplistic solutions' (Mullender, Everitt, Hardiker and Littlewood, 1993/4: 13). Some radical feminist and critical accounts of qualitative research methods have gone much further than this position, and have directed some of the criticism that has long been applied to quantitative research at traditional ethnography itself.

We believe that generalisations of this kind do not do justice to the challenge posed for social work and evaluating in practice by the epistemology and methodology of people working in the positivist traditions. Some writers working in these traditions have more recently conceded the limitations of a positivist approach. For example, Rotheray (1993), in a useful introductory overview, written in an irenic tone, accepts that a misleading 'pseudo-neutrality' marks the work of some positivists within social work. He also admits that the problem of a reductionist perspective on the meaning of social work is unavoidable in such studies and that positivism can have little to say about important issues of choice, free will and human responsibility. We will later raise serious reservations about present enthusiasm in some quarters for applications of positivist methodologies, especially in the field of work with offenders (see Chapter Nine). However, decisions about questions such as,

- should evaluating in practice be value-free?

- are methods of evaluating in practice different from those used in the natural sciences?, and

- do evaluation techniques objectify people and as a result serve the interests of the powerful at the expense of the poor?

have no necessary connection with whether one pursues, wittingly or otherwise, a positivist approach.

Paradigm talk also tends to subsume other related arguments which then become tarred with the same brush. For example, the major body of work accomplished by Karl Popper is almost entirely ignored by social workers. They are prone to neglect or to misread Popper's opposition to relativism and his thoroughgoing objectivism, as entailing a determinist worldview. Nothing could be further from Popper's position. His wholehearted anti-determinist stance was built on a belief that indeterminacy is an objective characteristic of the cosmos, and not just a product of our ignorance (Popper, 1979). For Popper, we are not constrained, determined and pushed by the past, but 'enticed' by the future. We do not live in a closed cosmos. His vision towards the close of his life was of 'the allure of the open future. The world is no longer a causal machine. It can now be seen to be an unfolding process, realising possibilities and unfolding new possibilities' (Popper, 1988). Social workers should pause if they are tempted to consign Popper - or positivism - to history's trash can.

Making ourselves accountable: reflexive and plausible practice

Evaluating in practice combines a particular cast of mind, a commitment to particular values and the assiduous cultivation of neglected practice antennae. This cast of mind requires a *reflexive* and *plausible* practice. All evaluations are produced with some audience in mind. They are social acts and socially validated, stemming from the fact that social workers are part and parcel of the setting, context and culture that they are trying to represent and evaluate. Dorothy Scott captures exactly the problem of a reflexive practice when she asks whether it is possible 'to look at the lens at the same time as one is looking through it' (Scott, 1989: 47).

The basic idea is not new to social work. Scott observes, for example, that countertransference is an instance of reflexivity. Some staff supervision models are also an attempt at reflexive work, and England's plea for appropriate description of practice stems in part from a recognition of ways in which practice can become reflexive. Some accounts of the client's self-understanding in counselling include pleas for *client* reflexivity (Howe, 1993: 132-134). Precisely because the participants in evaluating are part and parcel of the setting, we find our way back to the point that the story is shaped by the telling, and to tell the story is to 'restory' it. The more plausible the evaluating, the more probable that it will reflexively reconstitute the social reality it describes.

Reflexivity might seem a fairly unassuming cluster of ideas. However, there has been an acute radicalising of debate about reflexivity in the field of ethnography which, once adopted, fundamentally changes the purpose of evaluating in practice. An important criticism of positivism has been along the lines that people *make sense* of the world and that there are thus multiple and contingent realities rather than just one. Hammersley makes the telling point that 'such a view is not necessarily relativistic as it stands. However, it can become so if it is applied to social research itself' (Hammersley, 1995: 16). This is exactly what has taken place since the early 1970's, leading to a position which claims that knowledge, even the knowledge process, is without grounding or authority. 'Knowledge' itself is no longer the criterion, because all 'knowledge' claims are based on various assumptions (this development has been traced by Altheide and Johnson, 1994).

Once this thinking works its way through into questions of gender, race, disability and so on, the primary question for any evaluating in practice is no longer whether the social worker or even the service user understands problems more clearly. The purpose of evaluation now becomes whether service users have been *emancipated*. The external grounding for evaluating in practice thus comes to rest not in the process of claims to truth of some kind but 'rather in a commitment to a post-Marxism and a feminism with hope but no guarantees' (Lincoln and Denzin, 1994: 579). Evaluating in practice on this basis is not about reflective rigour in empowering but concerns a practice which is legitimated *only* through the test of whether it empowers and emancipates. 'Bias' is accepted and even embraced as a virtue. The test of validity is whose interests does that bias serve? (Hammersley, 1995: 42). Effectiveness *is* truth.

This question of what constitutes the external grounding of evaluating in practice leads us directly to the second requirement, *plausible* practice. What counted as sufficiently persuasive evidence of doing well or doing less well figured prominently in the social workers' accounts of their own evaluating in previous chapters of this book. The question, the consequences of which have far reaching influence on how practitioners evaluate, is whether such evaluating should be conducted mainly from an insider or outsider perspective.

We will consider first the essentially 'outsider' approach represented by the inference from Popper's argument that we should seek to falsify our evaluatings, and follow that with an example of an 'insider' approach to validating which takes as its starting point forms of analysis of narrative developed in the humanities rather than the sciences.

Popper told the story of how, early in his career, he visited the psychotherapist Alfred Adler in Vienna, who was distinguished for his work on developing the concept of the inferiority complex. Adler invited Popper to observe him at work in his consulting room, and later indicated that a person he had just seen exhibited the symptoms of an inferiority complex. Popper reports that he asked Adler how he knew this to be the case. 'Because of my thousand-fold experience', Adler apparently replied. The young Popper, too clever by half, we may be tempted to think, could not resist the retort, 'and now I suppose it is your thousand-and-one fold experience!'

Stories serve to make telling points. Popper's concern was that Adler's theorising was proceeding by searching for corroborating instances, and that this led it down the pathway of being ultimately unfalsifiable. This risk of adopting unfalsifiable hypotheses is sometimes illustrated in counselling approaches where the relationship between social worker and client is central to the therapeutic process. For example, defence mechanisms often take this form, so that a practitioner's hypothesis can be assumed to be confirmed whether or not the client agrees with the therapist. The very strength of a client's *resistance* to a practitioner's interpretation may be taken as indicative of the *validity* of that interpretation (Scott, 1989). The ideas of 'unconscious denial' and, in Marxist thinking, 'false consciousness' are alike in being illustrations of the Catch 22 of the unfalsifiable hypothesis. Concerns about 'false memory syndrome' illustrate how difficult this problem can prove in everyday practice. The opposing claims that therapists have been putting ideas into people's heads, and that children who have been abused face the double jeopardy of doubting social workers, will continue to be disputed partly because of the difficulty of falsifying either claim.

One commonsense understanding of falsification might proceed by saying that *theories* are always fallible, but the *empirical base* for theories is not fallible. Therefore falsification entails testing fallible theories with non-fallible facts. This was not Popper's position. As an anti-determinist he emphasised, even celebrated, the uncertainty of knowledge. Knowledge for Popper never equalled proven knowledge, because for him knowledge is not provable. When

Popper spoke of an empirical base, experimenting, observing, applying theories, and eliminating or falsifying theories, there were always at least invisible inverted commas around each word, indicating that they are fallible. Popper advocated all of these activities, but did so aware of the approximations to knowledge and of the fallibility and risk at every step in our conclusions. Exhortations to social workers elsewhere in this book to 'falsify' assume the same inverted commas. For example, when saying earlier in this chapter that social workers must describe practice in such a way that it renders access to and evaluation of its strengths and weaknesses feasible, we intend to say they must 'describe' their practice.

A vital conclusion follows. 'If a theory is falsified, it is proven false; if it is 'falsified' it may still be true' (Lakatos, 1970: 108). 'Eliminated' theories - and evaluations - may not be false. When social workers evaluate in practice, they are 'falsifying', not falsifying. This is very far from naive, dogmatic objectivism. Indeed, this may tempt us to drop out in the belief that testing our conclusions is meaningless. But Popper is severe on this point. In a memorable phrase he insists that our hypothesis 'must be made to stick its neck out.' But we must live with the uncertainty of what we know. We may reject an explanation but we cannot disprove it. The real debate is not whether social work is scientific but whether it is 'scientific'.

Illustration of the kinds of 'falsifying' questions social workers should ask include,

- Can we specify the circumstances under which we would be prepared to reject a particular explanation, or adherence to a certain practice model?

- What alternative explanations have we 'eliminated'?

- Does our practice tend to proceed by searches for corroborating, confirming instances?

- In what ways does the explanation we have adopted lead to novel 'facts' not following from rival explanations?

Social workers are unlikely to find this a comfortable approach. 'Falsifying' alternative explanations was rarely suggested by the practitioners to whom we spoke. The kind of falsification advocated by Popper provides an invaluable means of 'combining hard-hitting criticism with fallibilism' (Lakatos, 1970: 112) when evaluating our own practice. If evaluating in practice is to play a part at the heart of an empowering social work practice, it must be both critical and fallible.

This should not be read as a plea for falsification at any price. We saw earlier that England presents the apparently different criteria of 'plausibility' and 'adequacy' as the gauges against which practice should be evaluated. These 'shadow cousins' (Olesen, 1994: 163) of validity emerge when we locate social work closer to the humanities than to the sciences. What do we mean when we claim that an evaluating in practice narrative ought to be plausible? Freeman suggests that to be plausible a narrative ought to be *coherent* and *fitting*. By coherent he means that 'it ought to make sense of all the available information'. This does not mean that we will be able to resolve clearly every aspect of practice or that things sometimes are not quite senseless.

> All it means is that with some particular body of historical data at hand, the resultant narrative scheme ought to be able to encompass these data in a way that isn't fraught with obvious contradictions, stupidity and so forth.

In suggesting that a narrative should be fitting he concludes that, 'all things considered, the narrative ought to be able to make better sense than other possible narratives, whether actual or hypothetical' (Freeman, 1993: 163). This hermeneutically minded approach steers through the dilemma of wishing to avoid an objectivist position (the narrative reflects the way things really are), and yet recognises the common sense view that some interpretations and evaluating narratives are more plausible than others.

Freeman adds two riders which translate readily to social work evaluating. First, it is often the case that several interpretations appear not only equally coherent but equally plausible. Is there a way out of this impasse? 'The answer plainly is "No", and I'm afraid we will just have to live with this' (p165). Second, although plausibility is an important criterion, Freeman provides further sound advice for social workers, service users and audiences validating practice evaluatings.

> It is no less important that we...have an expansive enough idea of what constitutes plausibility as to be willing to stretch out our minds beyond the reach of the obvious. Stated another way, we must be receptive and respectful enough of the texts we encounter to remain open to the possibility of entirely new forms of interpretations: if the old plots won't do, then it might

be time to explore something different...a wholesale escape is out of the question. But stretching the boundaries of what is to be considered plausible is not. Do not confuse plausibility, then, with the superficial or the obvious, for it may be anything but that (p165).

We have already seen that to the radicalisation of reflexivity has been added a corresponding radicalisation of validity. A frequently advocated view is that validity depends on the audiences and that validity will be quite different for different audiences. 'No permanent telling of a story can be given. There are only different versions of different, not the same, stories' (Denzin, 1994: 506). From this viewpoint validity does not depend on demonstrating the adequacy with which the world has been represented, but the extent to which the product serves a political usefulness. The expression 'catalytic validity' captures closely this political meaning of validity measured by the degree to which evaluation or research empowers and emancipates. There are, in consequence, frequent references in the ethnography literature to crises of representation and legitimation. If the evaluation process is itself relative, then can we ever hope to speak authentically of the experience of another person? I believe we can.

A plausible and falsifying evaluating in practice must, in our view, start from five criteria of validity (Altheide and Johnson, 1994). Taken together, these criteria require a reflexive account of evaluating in practice which lays open to audience understanding the processes by which practitioners and service users accomplished their evaluating.

First, the *substance* of evaluatings in practice should display a demonstrable approximation to the real world. Value-free knowledge is, of course, a chimera. But it does not follow that it is may not remain in some senses normative (MacKay, 1987, 1988). Validity 'represents the always just out of reach, but answerable, claim' made for the authority of the evaluation (Lincoln and Denzin, 1994: 579).

Second, the *relationships* between the social worker, the service users and carers are an inseparable dimension of evaluation. The more the audience can symbolically engage with the social worker about the host of routinely encountered problems that compromise evaluating in practice, the more our confidence in the plausibility of that evaluation increases. The question is not whether issues of trust, mistakes, the role of the social worker, the type of evidence, or the interpretations of practice were *problems*, but whether they were *treated* as problems?

Third, evaluating in practice must make clear the *perspective* from which the evidence is interpreted. The ethical pluralism that marks social work makes it particularly apposite that social workers should be required to specify the purposes of practice and its evaluation, so that audiences are able to recognise the 'signature' and have an honest statement of what they are being asked to buy.

The fourth and fifth criteria require reflexive accounts of the actual and intended *audiences* of the evaluation and openness about the *style* of any final product. Work in the humanities has drawn helpful attention to the different criteria of plausibility and adequacy that follow from different literary *genres*. For instance, a plausible report to a *case conference* may not be plausible as a basis for adequate exchanges about the same person between *colleagues*. We thus encounter the recognition that evaluating, recording and writing about that evaluation are overlapping activities.

Whoever evaluates clinical practice needs to tell 'method-ologically, rhetorically and clinically convincing stories' (Miller and Crabtree, 1994: 348). A methodologically convincing story will tell how the evaluation was arrived at. What were the relationships between evaluator and other participants? What are the relationships with the audiences? What is the evaluator's intent? A rhetorically convincing story will answer how believable the account is. It 'assures the reader that the author has walked in their shoes' (p348). Finally, does this evaluation make clinical sense? Therefore, evaluating in practice will be convincing

> if the methods are appropriate for the question, and the investigator's relationship with informants, data and audience are clearly addressed; if the audience recognises itself in the findings; and if the question and results matter to clinical participants (p349).

We have argued that evaluating in practice exercises a 'disciplined subjectivity' which starts from the tacit knowing in action which is a feature of all professional practice. It's defining elements are:

- its *purpose* is evaluating *for* service users

- its *process* involves

    - participatory evaluating *with* service users

    - reflecting on tacit knowing-in-practice

–   describing practice in ways that render access to its strengths and weaknesses feasible

–   mutual reflexivity of both practitioner and service user

–   legitimation through falsifying and grounded plausibility

This model of evaluating in practice draws on developments in the epistemology and methodology of ethnography, the growing influence of the humanities on the social sciences, recent work on participatory research in Third World development understanding and practice, and Donald Schon's work on the nature of professional inquiry.   It retains belief in the possibility of a grounded realism and a commit-ment to 'falsifying' social work explanations, evaluatings and action proposals.   In the final part of this chapter we will review the remaining elements of this model, and weigh up what is entailed in evaluating with and for service.

Evaluating for and with service users

Recent debates about the validity and plausibility of research in the literature and practice of qualitative social science impart, as we have already seen, a sharp twist to questions about the purpose and process of evaluating in practice.   Is good evaluating in practice useful because it is true or true because it is useful?   The traditional view has been based on the belief that understanding is ultimately useful, even if in some unknown or unknowable sense, and on an acceptance that investigations should sometimes concentrate on issues of political relevance.   But commitment to the values of any one group has conventionally been ruled out.   We do not believe this position is workable as a basis for evaluating in social work practice.

We have already seen how arguments for user involvement in evaluation have entered social work through the requirements of community care legislation.   'As the commitment to user involvement develops, researchers need to find a variety of ways in which people can feel part of the research' (Barnes, 1992: 16).   At the very least 'the reflective practitioner...attributes to his client, as well as to himself, a capacity to mean, know and plan.   He...tries to discover the limits of his expertise through reflective conversation with the client' (Schon, 1983: 295-6).   Calls for participatory evaluation have come from many quarters, including user involvement initiatives, self-help and advocacy groups (Adams, 1990) and community development groups (eg Meadows and Turkie, 1988). We will illustrate the strength and range of these arguments through brief outlines of feminist and Third World development pleas for politically committed, participatory evaluation.

Early appeals for participatory evaluation drew their strength from a traditional, redistributive welfare position. Holman pleads for 'research from the underside' because, 'the values I hold are such that I long for the end of poverty and the promotion of equality. My interest in research is just this, how can research help the poor?' (Holman, 1987: 669). He criticises much otherwise good poverty research as being *about* rather than *by* or *with* the poor, and hopes that,

> Research from the underside might even stimulate the socially deprived to agitate more forcibly for a lowering of the standards of the wealthy as well as for an improvement of those of the poor (p682).

Although he holds that research from the underside does not exclude the involvement of research experts, Holman proposes a 'bottom-up model in which the investigated become the investigators' (p680), and whose effectiveness is judged by whether,

i	they (the poor) define the issues to be researched;
ii	they contribute to deciding how the topic should be researched;
iii	they participate in collecting the research material;
iv	they interpret the findings;...
v	the research enables both practitioners and respondents to be more fully aware of the issues being investigated;
vi	the poor use the research findings for their own purposes (p672).

Feminist evaluating

Feminist work on research methodology has pervasive implications for evaluating in practice. Although there are important variations on issues of epistemology within feminism (Hawkesworth, 1989), all feminist positions start from the proposition that when evaluating practice, the practitioner must ask questions which make sense within women's experience, and must evaluate practice *for* women. Most feminists would reject the idea that there is one single, woman's experience. Third World, black and lesbian feminisms have together served to 'dissolve the conceptualisation of 'woman'' (Olesen, 1994:

160). This creates obvious problems for feminists who wish to argue that women's experiences are more reliable than men's. However, many feminists reject a relativist approach to practice knowledge, often basing their case on feminist standpoint theory. Standpoint theory has its origins in Marxist and Hegelian arguments that reality is obscured to people from certain backgrounds because of the effects of ideology. For Marx, the way in which the proletariat could escape ideology's grip was through the possession of privileged access to a form of understanding not available to other classes. Applied to social work,

> Standpoint theory builds on the assertion that the less powerful members of society experience a different reality as a consequence of their oppression...To survive they must have knowledge, awareness and sensitivity of both the dominant group's view of society and their own - the potential for 'double vision' or consciousness - and thus the potential for a more complete view of social reality'
>
> (Swigonski, 1993: 173).

The theory makes two linked assertions, the double vision of the oppressed and the partial vision of the more powerful - 'privilege and its invisibility to those who hold it' (p174).

What implications does this position have for how social workers evaluate their direct practice? First, it values an 'epistemological egalitarianism' and espouses - if such a politically shaky verb may be used - an emphasis on personal experience as providing 'a more complete view of social reality' than scientific method. Feminists often reject dualist distinctions such as culture-nature, objective-subjective, and public-private on the grounds that they each have masculine-feminine layered over them. This belief that reason is itself gendered is often associated with a rejection of quantitative methods. 'Equation of quantification with objectivity has been critiqued by feminist scholars who point out that quantification has its own inherent biases and distortions' (Cook and Fonnow, 1990: 77).

Second, standpoint theory also entails a model of evaluation, which works 'towards the participation of members of oppressed groups in every phase of research activity' (Swigonski, 1993: 178). This model is linked to a belief that hierarchical relationships are unacceptable among women, and that truth will only be discovered through non-hierarchical relationships.

Thirdly, an 'activist' view of evaluation as 'undertaken for explicitly political purposes' (Swigonski, 1993: 181) is often associated with standpoint theory. It involves helping members of oppressed groups gain political consciousness. Cook and Fonnow say that 'the research process itself can become a process of "conscientisation" for both the researcher and the subjects of research,' thus 'encouraging politicisation and activism on the part of research subjects.' They conclude that 'the most thorough kind of knowledge and understanding comes through efforts to change social phenomena' (pp 75, 80).

Finally, standpoint theory is committed to empowerment. We should 'evaluate up' not 'evaluate down', to adapt a phrase from Sandra Harding. Research is for 'the empowerment and social transformation of clients...Research, practice and social action are one unified effort. The empowerment of oppressed groups and of practitioner-researchers occurs simultaneously' (Swigonski, 1993: 181-2). In a much quoted comment, Cook and Fonnow say, "The purpose of knowledge is to change or transform patriarchy...Description without an eye for transformation is inherently conservative" (1990: 79).

Standpoint theory has not been without its critics (Hawkesworth, 1989; Hammersley, 1995), especially on the grounds that its claims to truth are unconvincing. To Mary Hawkesworth the idea of a privileged female perspective 'appears to be highly implausible'. 'Given the diversity and fallibility of all human knowers, there is no good reason to believe that women are any less prone to error, deception or distortion than men' (1989: 544). The appeal to experience or intuitive knowledge she finds equally unpersuasive. 'Intuition provides a foundation for claims about the world that is at once authoritarian, admitting no further discussion, and relativist, since no individual can refute another's "immediate" apprehension of reality' (p545).

Ethical problems and doubts regarding whether it is possible to have a feminist ethnography are another area of active debate. Stacey wonders 'whether the appearance of greater respect for and equality with research subjects in the ethnographic approach masks a deeper, more dangerous form of exploitation' (Stacey, 1988: 22). She describes two instances from her research. In one case a lesbian woman became a 'fundamentalist Christian' and in the other a woman who had left the researcher with hours of tape material died. In both of these examples she concludes that 'conflicts of interest between the ethnographer as authentic, related person (ie participant), and as exploiting researcher (ie observer)' are 'an inescapable feature of the ethnographic method' (p23). The greater the apparent mutuality of the relationship between qualitative evaluator and service user, the greater the danger that the method will expose people to exploitation. She suggests that feminists tend to suffer the 'delusion of alliance', whereas, in deciding what to include in her report regarding the lesbian and Christian woman, 'whatever we decide, my ethnography will betray a feminist principle' (p24).

It is clear that these questions of epistemology and of ethics pose serious issues for feminists - and non-feminists - who engage in qualitative evaluating in practice of the kind advocated in this book. There is no obvious solution, though there are two guidelines that should, in our view, characterise feminist evaluating in practice. First, feminists should consider whether partial truths and reduced claims should mark their practice. Hawkesworth insists that it is quite possible to 'distinguish between partial views (the inescapable condition of human cognition) and false beliefs, superstitions, irrebutable presumptions, wilful distortions' (1989: 553); and Stacey concludes that feminists can only aim for partial feminist ethnographies. Second, feminists should explore the 'difficult contradictions between feminist principles and ethnographic research' and evaluating (Stacey, 1988: 22). Feminists 'need not assert that theirs is the only or final word on complex questions' (Hawkesworth, 1989: 555). In making women's lives problematic feminist social workers 'should not turn away from rendering their own practices problematic' (Olesen, 1994: 169).

Participatory evaluation

Arguments for participatory, advocacy evaluation, which are at least as significant as those advanced by feminist writers, have been put forward by practitioners working in the field of Third World development. From the mid 1970s Non-Governmental Organisations (NGOs) such as Oxfam and Save the Children were a major force in a changing view of development practice which aimed to 'include the poor people themselves in the process of problem identification and project implementation and evaluation' (Cervinskas, 1991: 27). A central objective of participatory research is 'the enhancement of the ability of the poor to generate and control their own knowledge, and control the means of the production of knowledge' (p32), and hence it is 'a vehicle for understanding and changing the world simultaneously' (Edwards, 1989: 128). The focus is on collective inquiry about concrete problems, mutual collaboration and action for change, and the methods borrow from popular education and community traditions of self-help.

Although initial enthusiasm has been tempered somewhat by the difficulties of securing authentic participation, participatory research challenges social work evaluating at a number of points. For example, there has been a helpful debate among development activists about the relationship between grassroots participation and change at the macro levels. The collapse of some structuralist theories of society in the late 1980s made this question especially acute (eg Booth, 1994). In a later paper Edwards insists that we need not require all inquiry to be participatory. However, while work at higher levels cannot easily be participatory, 'to be relevant, research must *in some way* be linked to the real experience and concerns of people at grassroots level' (1994: 284). 'Scaling up' the impact of evaluation becomes a crucial task. Edwards also answers the criticism that participatory research may lead to knowledge which is useful to the sorts of causes we disapprove of rather than those of which we approve (cf Rossi, 1987). He does not duck this problem. 'By its very nature the process of empowerment is uncertain...the ultimate destination is unknown' (1994: 288).

Participatory research is not free from problems (Cervinskas, 1991). For example, the risk of 'participant manipulation', parallel to the ethical issue about feminist ethnography raised by Stacey, is difficult to overcome, partly because initiatives for projects tend to come from 'experts'. In addition there is a concern about participatory research being taken over and co-opted by Western academics and practitioners. Yet mainline development academics have admitted that their work does not altogether escape the strictures of criticism from Edwards and others. I reject Third Worldism - the belief that the study of less-developed countries needs special methods (Shaw and Al-Awwad, 1994) - and am convinced that social workers have much to learn from the efforts of those who wrestle with the needs and rights of distant strangers. Yet participatory evaluation offers a sharply uncomfortable perspective on social work practice, especially when applied to community interventions.

Insider and outsider

If evaluating in practice ought to be marked by mutual reflexivity, falsification, a search for grounded plausibility and a commitment to evaluating for and with the service user, then the social worker must hold to the twin, uncomfortable realities that understanding comes by change and change comes by understanding. The Gordian knot cannot be cut by dropping either change or understanding from the equation. Dannie Abse's poem at the head of this chapter about his own role as both 'white coat' doctor and 'purple coat' poet is apposite. Evaluating in practice encompasses, for all participants, being both insider and outsider, member and stranger, white coat evaluator and purple coat practitioner. It demands the cultivation of 'anthropological strangeness' (Lofland, 1971) and the avoidance of sentimentality, which we are guilty of

> when we refuse, for whatever reason, to investigate some matter that should properly be regarded as problematic. We are sentimental, especially, when our reason is that we would prefer not to know what is going on, if to know would be to violate some sympathy whose existence we may not even be aware of
>
> (Becker, 1970: 132-3).

Service users with whom we engage in evaluating are faced with learning a new language, and are simultaneously onlookers in the stalls and a member of the cast (the metaphor is from Schutz, 1971: 97). Even when participation and partnership appear most genuine, service users may miss the 'fringes' of the language of organisations, the secondary meanings derived from the context, and the private codes derived from past experience they do not share.

The role of the practitioner is different but not more simple. She is inescapably working at the boundaries between the citizen and the state (Henderson, Jones and Thomas 1980), a stranger to the service user for whom the meeting with the social worker or community worker (Rees, 1974; Thomas, 1975) is often 'no more than contact'. Evaluating in practice may threaten the freedom of the service user not to reveal. Through research and evaluating we create the anxiety in others that 'someone knows'. Donald Warwick warned some time ago of the risk that we may 'reinforce the tendency of individuals to be wary and to live for the record' (Warwick, 1982: 52). Evaluating in practice consumes resources of money and personnel but also of goodwill and tolerance. These resources are finite. An evaluation-minded practitioner must make sure her clients do not become footnotes to her favourite thesis. We have the obligation to evaluate sensitive topics with service users, but we do not have the right to deceive, exploit or manipulate. Evaluating in practice cannot countenance what Robert Merton called 'sociological sadism'.

Evaluating in practice cannot avoid the criteria of practical and political relevance. Evaluating is not ethnography, and social work is more than evaluating. The uncertainty of knowledge is no excuse for inaction. Such inaction assumes too strong a relationship between the truth of a belief and the practical consequences of acting on it. Reid's question from a different context will bear repeating. 'Is it better to make limited but well documented progress or to work towards more important goals with less certainty of what we have attained?' (Reid, 1988: 45). But social workers should pick their targets and beware of chronic commitment and activism. An evaluating that is not seen to be falsifying and anti-sentimental will rapidly lose any relevance it originally enjoyed. Hammersley's warning against the anti-racist version of activist research and evaluation is persuasive.

> Anti-racists are unwise to reject the conventional model of research in favour of the activist conception. One reason for this is that the propaganda capacity of research is to a large extent parasitical upon the conventional model. Once research becomes seen as geared to the pursuit of particular political goals, with research results being selected, even in part, according to their suitability for propaganda purposes, its propaganda value is gone
> (Hammersley, 1993: 444).

Hammersley has become very controversial at this point, but he provides a reminder of the inevitable tension for the evaluator in practice between their insider and outsider roles. In the next three chapters we will describe ways in which a qualitative evaluating in practice can be developed, while keeping in mind the challenges to values, skills, knowledge and understanding that all evaluating will present.

7 New agenda, new methods: evaluating assessments and plans

You walk into the room
With your pencil in your hand
You see somebody naked
And you say, 'Who is that man?'
You try so hard
But you don't understand
Just what you'll say
When you get home

Because something is happening here
But you don't know what it is
Do you, Mister Jones?

Bob Dylan ('*Ballad of a Thin Man*')

We assess people as soon as they come through the door.

Social worker

All social work is assessment.

Social work manager

Assessment and planning predominate in almost every social work method and setting. They are, in one practitioner's words, 'the lifeblood of the profession.' The development of agreement based social work in community care and social work with children and their carers has probably had the effect of further increasing local authority social workers' preoccupation with planning. The development of Home Office National Standards may well have had a similar impact on the work of probation officers.

We are not sure that these developments will have uniformly beneficial repercussions for the quality of assessing and planning activities in social work. The growth of management by measurement and accountability does, as we have argued in Chapter Five, have its downside in terms of the likely consequences for the quality of practice. A respected commentator on the American scene has gone as far as to conclude that 'there is no question that assessment as we have known it is waning in social work practice.' She lays the blame for this at the door of 'the accountability mania, the rush to quantification and the general anti-intellectualism of our times' (Meyer, 1992: 303). Concern has also been voiced about the 'demise of thorough assessment in the Probation Service' (MacDonald, 1994: 415).

Evidence about older people and children and families' experience of using agreement based social work practice reveals three difficult problems. There is an almost universal assumption by social workers that they already have an agreement with clients. 'It is part of the professional clothing to assume that the work is based on negotiation and consent' (Fisher, 1983: 48). They therefore see little reason to consider changing their practice. Second, the agreements that have existed are usually in the form of an understanding. They are verbal rather than written and are often rather nonspecific. Finally, there is a reluctance to allow clients freedom to define their own problems. Fears are expressed by practitioners that to give primacy to user-defined problems could be deskilling for social workers.

A further reason why it is difficult to generalise about assessment and planning is that there are wide differences in the character and time devoted to these activities by social workers. The purchaser-provider split, the exercise of statutory functions, and the fact that some agencies are better resourced than others are only some of the most obvious reasons for such differences. If practitioners believe they have few resources for intervention then investment of time and effort in assessment may seem wasted effort that raises false expectations. In addition, some social workers are unlikely to place more than minimal stress on assessments and plans because they fear this will disempower service users and lead to them being acted on as the subjects of professional decision making. Practitioners in direct access homelessness agencies and most women's aid refuges probably adopt this position.

Even within larger, more structured agencies, assessment and planning decisions will not be treated in a uniform manner, for a wide variety of reasons. The style, content and process of assessment will vary. Some kinds of assessment may be 'sub-contracted' to specialist partner agencies, particularly if they are seen as requiring a higher level of interpretive skills. The boundaries between assessment and intervention will also be blurred, perhaps particularly in short-term interventions where assessment may be regarded as simultaneous with intervention. In early research fieldwork from which the social work quotations at the head of this chapter are taken, practitioners sometimes made a working distinction between formal and informal assessment. It is in the informal sense that all social work is assessment. In formal assessment it is likely that some kind of written product will be required. Scott implies a possible explanation of the differences between informal and formal assessment when she points out that 'the social worker is immersed in a continuous process of naturalistic inquiry.' Yet the practitioner is 'perhaps typically reframing it in a more linear way in the written form of assessment.' If this is the case then 'the classic texts on casework...may not reflect the reality of practice' (Scott, 1989: 40).

We saw in the previous chapter that medical practitioners engage in decision taking processes that are largely specific to the specialist when they make routine decisions (Bloor, 1978). It seems probable that similar diversity will exist within social work, thus contributing still further to a lack of uniformity in decision making. Assessments may also operate as a variety of claims making, intended either to ration or to acquire areas of work. Assessments should not, therefore, be regarded as simply technical tasks of information gathering and agreed professional inference. An example of assessment operating as claims making is implied in one social work manager's perception of a specialist team elsewhere in the same agency that, 'the reason they carry out assessments is because they do not trust our assessments.'

Notwithstanding these changes and problems, assessment and planning will remain at the leading edge of social work practice. In this chapter we search for promising ingredients of competence in evaluating assessment and planning in practice. Competencies, of course, not in the sense of technical skills, but as 'the practical application of values and principles without which activities are unlikely to be effective or satisfactory' (CCETSW, 1995: 25). Our model of evaluating in practice rules out of court strongly empiricist and reductionist evaluations or at least pushes them to the fringes. But our concern in these next three chapters is not primarily to warn off but to stimulate an expansive mood, to sensitise social workers' methodological antennae, and push practitioners to be purposeful and opportunist evaluators in practice.

Perhaps the main assumption behind these following chapters is that social workers' practice has been woefully impoverished by their reliance on a narrow routine of ways of learning about service users. True, there has been a broadening of ways of working. Social-skills methods, and cognitive approaches in work with offenders, have led to new practice tactics, and the range of therapeutic interventions in clinical settings and some residential units is steadily widening. But most social workers probably regard these and other innovations as specialist or minority activities. Even when we do experiment with new methods, we typically do not think of them in terms of how they might enrich our evaluation.

The case for evaluating in practice is a case for work which permeates every aspect of practice. The process framework of these following chapters is intended to make that very point. Not that a simple process line of assess, plan, intervene and conclude is all that meaningful. Even when social work seems, to either service user or practitioner, to fall into identifiable phases, these will overlap, lack order and sequence and vary greatly in length. For example, an elderly persons' home, an emergency duty team, a refuge for women, or a probation team will each identify and weight phases differently. Furthermore, in some settings it may make sense to think of maintenance as a phase, or even, despite all we have said, as evaluation. So the fact that, for instance, we have something to say about the potential of participant observation methods later in *this* chapter rather than in the next chapter is simply that the majority of the applications that came to mind were assessment oriented in their main thrust. Our location of life-course methods in this chapter or focus groups in the following may perhaps seem equally arbitrary.

We should remove one other possible source of mis-understanding, arising from talk about 'methods'. We have said that we see evaluating in practice as a way of accomplishing change through understanding. It will usually be clear from the context when we use 'method' in the conventional social work sense of a particular way of working, and when we intend to convey 'method' as a way of understanding-for-change.

Evaluating assessing and planning in practice

Evaluation and assessment are distinct yet inextricable. We observed the tendency of social workers in the accounts recorded earlier to elide assessment, planning, review and appraisal with evaluation. In our view this is an unhelpful strategy. It narrows evaluating in practice to one phase of practice, risks routinising evaluating by tying it to formal procedures required by agencies, associates it too closely with 'Evaluation with a Capital E', and exonerates practitioners from evaluating once the initial phase of involvement is negotiated. Unfortunately this muddying of the waters is often encouraged by guidance and standards required of practitioners. For example, the Home Office National Standards for probation officers tend to use evaluation and assessment interchangeably. When *'evaluating'* the seriousness of offences, the report writer is told to *'consider'* the seriousness of the offences and that 'such *assessment'* need not be lengthy. *'Evaluating* seriousness' is also described elsewhere in the Standards as *'Assessment* of Seriousness'.

We try to avoid this confusion. In order to evaluate, social work must be subject to a description and analysis which can determine its quality. It has to be described in such a way that it makes access to its strengths and weaknesses feasible. 'Without adequate description there can be no possibility of evaluation' (England, 1986: 155). If we are to reach a position where we have plausibly and adequately helped, then the links between understanding, action and effect - assessment, intervention and outcome - must be made clear. Schon's conclusion is that reflective practitioners judge their problem setting in the light of questions such as, Can I solve the problem I have set? Do I like what I get when I solve this problem? Have I made the situation coherent? Have I made it congruent with my fundamental values and theories? Have I kept inquiry moving? (Schon, 1983).

The social workers whose accounts appeared in the earlier part of this book often referred to the absence of clear assessments, plans and objectives when they tried to explain why work had not gone well. The lack of a workable plan 'to get me there' had led to aimless, wandering intervention. 'If we haven't got anything to *start* with we're *bound* to get lost.' Aimless intervention is 'just too trivialising.' The problem does not get 'unlocked', practice becomes 'all surface containment', and the service user's situation may become yet worse as a direct outcome of social work involvement.

Evaluating in practice for assessment and planning must address the *agenda* and the *methodology* of practice, and it is these two themes that we will focus on through the main part of this chapter.

Evaluating assessment and planning agenda

Social workers are insiders, with all the unexpected disadvantages that being an insider brings. Assessment and planning too easily miss the 'peculiar combination of nearness and remoteness, concern and indifference' which Simmel defined well as the objectivity of the stranger, with its ability to see patterns that the insider may not see (quoted Collins, 1986).

Assessments of 'labelling', for example, sometimes serve as a convenient myth which closes down rather than opens up the possibility of reflexive evaluating. Despite the criticisms of labelling theory that have appeared in the literature on deviance, social workers may too quickly allege labelling of their clients as if once asserted, the reality has been demonstrated. Emerson long ago pointed out in her discussion of responses to deviant behaviour that labelling may not be very easy to 'catch' after all. Labelling results from the application of a set of procedures for assessing situations and deciding how to proceed. The process of assessing involves negotiations over which framework of rules to apply, in order to decide whether behaviour is rule-breaking. Emerson argued that these negotiation processes often involve ambiguity, where the situation is familiar to the professional insider and unfamiliar to the service user. This may be especially likely to occur if the service user is a newcomer. The more that the unfamiliar stranger rejects the social worker's conceptual schemes about deviance - for example, by insisting that they did not intend to break a rule - the more the assessment and planning situation will be thrown into confusion and left to *ad hoc* negotiations. Negotiations act as structural inhibitions against labelling by providing the opportunity for persons to elude labelling and secure a stance from the social worker that 'nothing unusual is happening' (Emerson, 1970).

An observational study of clients using a maternal and child health centre also provides an illustration of how the assessment situation may be more complex and less self-evident than social workers on the inside may assume. The difference was very apparent of child management styles of mothers from different social class backgrounds who used the centre. 'The middle-class mothers appeared liberal to the point of permissiveness in their limit setting, while the lower-class mothers appeared authoritarian and punitive' (Scott, 1989: 41). A traditional social work explanation would rest on the surface and draw conclusions about class differences in child rearing behaviour.   Yet interviews with the mothers in their own homes revealed that the extreme differences noted in the centre were far less obvious, and both groups of mothers were anxious to present themselves as 'good mothers' according to what they perceived to be the nurse's expectations.   Scott concludes that this is best interpreted in terms of the meaning of the *agency* to the mothers.   Each group of mothers regarded the clinic as 'a stage on which they felt some pressure to act out the role of good mother.'   But,

> For the middle-class mothers, being a good mother in their own eyes and those of the nurse meant being liberal and child centred in their child-rearing style.   For the lower-class mothers, being a good mother meant having children who could behave properly in a public place (p42).

The effect of the illustrations from Emerson and Scott is to demand of social workers a meticulous search for negative cases, for differences rather than for confirmations.   Does someone else - a colleague, another professional, a service user - make a different assessment with the same 'evidence'?   Are our accounts of fairly stable things, such as ability levels or chronic illness effects, different at different times?   Does our assessment lead to 'accurate' predictions, or at least to better predictions than rival explanations, for example, from colleagues who work within a different practice framework?   Recalling Popper, the inverted commas matter.   Social workers cannot make accurate predictions from evidence, but only provisional and less certain 'accurate' predictions from 'evidence'.   Orienting practice assessments to falsification does not, of course, trap practice in a stereotypical positivism.   This is because falsification does not belong only to quantitative strategies.   Qualitative evaluation, particularly the empirical variety linked with grounded theory approaches, also locates falsification at the heart of strategies for achieving adequate explanation (eg Glaser and Strauss, 1967; Corbin and Strauss, 1990; Strauss and Corbin, 1990).

A moment ago we cast the social worker in the role of insider. Feminist standpoint theory would, of course, counter this, starting as it does from the position that women share the double vision of the oppressed.   They are 'the outsider within' (Collins, 1986).   Black feminist research has emphasised the multiple and interlocking effects of being black and being a woman, and has demonstrated the importance of black women's culture and the self-definition of black women.   For black women in social work, outsider within status will always generate tensions.

People who become outsiders within are forever changed by their new status...Outsiders within occupy a special status - they become different people, and their difference sensitises them to patterns that may be more difficult for established...insiders to see

(Collins, 1986: S29).

There are three basic responses that black women in social work can adopt to this status. They may seek to resolve the tension by leaving and remaining outsiders. Alternatively they may choose to suppress their difference by striving to become 'thinking as usual' social work insiders. Both of these choices rob social work of its diversity and weaken its identity. The most difficult choice is to encourage and institutionalise outsider-within ways of seeing. Patricia Collins is talking about black women within sociology but her conclusions apply with similar force to social work. Black women must 'learn to trust their own personal and cultural biographies as significant sources of knowledge' (p.S29) and bring these ways of knowing back into social work, so that they are free to be different and to challenge.

A feminist evaluating of assessment and planning will draw on a set of questions in which women's experiences are the test of the adequacy of what is said and planned - the test of the concepts used, the way information is gathered, and how it is interpreted and organised. Question such as, do assessment questions make sense within women's experiences? Concerns about why particular images of women are assumed in forms of provision or in sentences available to the courts are one illustration of how this question has helped reframe practitioners' agenda for service planning. The practice of peer evaluation and 'gatekeeping', described by a probation officer earlier in this book, has been discussed as a means of anti-discriminatory assessment practice in work with child sexual abusers and in the mental health field as well as in probation practice (Waterhouse, Dobash and Carnie, 1995; Gregg-Scott, Jowett and Morgan, 1993; Broad, 1994). Are social work assessments and plans *for* women? Do they provide answers for women or only for welfare or justice agencies? Are assessments and plans reflexive? For instance, participatory evaluation methods will incorporate some possibility for 'assessing up', through women service users evaluating the actions of practitioners.

Can men do feminist social work? Women working from a feminist standpoint theory would probably conclude that men can make feminist assessments and plans so long as women's experiences are the adequacy test for problems, for the information collected and explanations, so long as plans are made *for* women (Harding, 1987). Feminist writers in social work have sometimes taken a more moderating position. Drawing from the work of Gilligan on female and male voices, Davis' aim is to find 'ways to allow both voices to speak and of hearing both as speaking valued, albeit different, truths' (Davis, 1985: 111). Women's voice is embedded in connectedness with others. It assumes the primacy of relationship, and is expressed in an ethic of care. Women develop a model of thinking that is 'contextual and narrative'. Thus the use and valuation of intuition is implicit in the voice of women. Women's voice acknowledges the essential inequalities in the world and holds responsibility for others, and thus women are likely to judge themselves is terms of their ability to care. From childhood girls sacrifice their games to maintain relationships.

Men's voice is embedded in separateness from others. It speaks of autonomy and independence, and has an ethic of justice. It speaks of assuming responsibility first for oneself. The characteristic model of thinking is abstract and formal, and for men there are clear solutions. From childhood onwards boys' games teach them to sacrifice relationships for rules.

Davis views the growth of assessment instruments and contracts as indicative of a desire to replace the female by the male voice in social work. She welcomes contracts insofar as they correct for the practice of social workers trying to fulfil their own agendas unknown to the clients; but she warns against the way

> they also protect the worker from feeling a responsibility to take care of the client and protect the client from being taken care of by the worker. Thus, contracts provide a 'safe' connection between worker and client, protecting the autonomy of each
>
> (Davis, 1985: 110).

The argument that women's view is privileged, has had to take on board the differentiating effects of criticisms from women with disabilities, women from the Third World, black and lesbian women (eg Whitmore, 1994). We have already said that - along with some feminist writers and practitioners - we are not happy with all aspects of feminist standpoint theory (pp 119-120). Becker's warning of the danger of sentimentality, of refusing for whatever reason to investigate some matter that should properly be regarded as problematic, is also one that cuts across feminist standpoint claims to privileged knowledge. We noticed in the previous chapter that some feminists have warned that, in making women's lives problematic, feminists 'should not turn away from making their own practices problematic' (Olesen, 1994: 169), and they need to be aware of the potential contradictions in feminist ethnography which can lead to those methods being as worrisome as those of quantitative researchers.

The hazard of sentimentality in setting assessment and planning agenda also raises its head when social workers are operating in the field of rhetoric and claims making. This is less commonly the case in working with individuals and families and more likely to happen when social workers are involved in service or project development tasks. Social workers are on both the receiving and making ends of rhetorical claims: the family, AIDS, drugs, homelessness, criminal justice legislation, rape, domestic violence, ritual abuse - the list of grounds for claims is almost endless. Social workers often display appropriate scepticism of rhetoric by others, but not always of their own or of that which originates from 'sympathetic' groups, whether they be Shelter, the Big Issue, the Howard League, or the Terence Higgins Trust. Assuming social workers do not want to be involved in cynical claims, then sentimental claims rhetoric needs avoiding.

The agenda becomes clearer if we consider the process by which a social problem becomes recognised as such. Social workers need to be good claims makers, and to learn from successful claims. A commonsense, objectivist definition of a social problem is that it is an undesirable social condition. Best (1989) points out that this neglects the subjective dimensions, in that a social problem is such because people believe it to be. Child abuse, for instance, may come to be regarded as a social problem without anyone needing to demonstrate that a new social condition has emerged. A constructionist perspective focuses on the processes by which people designate some condition as a social problem. So social problems refer to two very different things in each perspective. For the objectivist social problems are *social conditions*. For the social constructionist social problems are claims making *activities*, and the social conditions are of little interest in their own right.

In practice the constructionist position is more varied than this in that its advocates often assume that they possess some background knowledge of actual social conditions. In response to this mixture of social condition and claim, Best advocates what he describes as 'contextual constructionism', which recognises the importance of the process by which claims are made; but he also argues that any claim can be evaluated against social conditions. For example, whereas strict constructionists would treat values as a resource for making claims, contextual constructionists would recognise that values may be the cause of claims makers' behaviour (Best, 1987). This position, which focuses on both the medium and the message of claims making, appears to be one which allows self-aware evaluation of social workers' own claims and also an agenda of critical questions by which to appraise the claims of others.

Child prostitution provides an illustration. Those who practice and research in the field are divided on whether to emphasise the direct impact of childhood experience of sexual abuse as a cause of later involvement in prostitution, or the effect of leaving home and being without shelter.   Each of these approaches is used to support different investments in service provision.   Service and project development will hinge on the definition of the problem, estimates of its scale, claims regarding trends and underlying warrants which justify action. Because the population of young people involved in prostitution is inevitably hidden, aspects of any claim will always be disputable. The extent and character of rough sleeping poses similar questions. Policy makers may define rough sleeping to include those who *choose* to leave accommodation, just as the definition of child prostitutes as 'runaways' underscores the apparent volitional aspects of the behaviour. A strong emphasis on volition may be used as a 'reason' for limiting the extent of response. Claims about the extent of either problem stem directly from the kind of definition adopted in the first place. Rossi, a liberal, reformist academic researcher, was vociferously attacked and ostracised by advocacy communities in Chicago for his research on rough sleeping in the city, which produced an estimate only about one-tenth of the estimate used by the Chicago Coalition for the Homeless (Rossi, 1987). 'The major theme was that our report had seriously damaged the cause of the homeless people in Chicago by providing state and local officials with an excuse to dismiss the problem as trivial' (p79). Such issues are not straightforward to resolve, but must be addressed if social workers' claims making is to effectively influence agenda setting.

Evaluating assessment and planning methodology

Challenging and shaping the *agenda* of evaluating in practice makes heavy demands. Yet even if we suppose from what we have said in the first part of this chapter that social workers *can* have some impact on the agenda of assessment and planning, evaluating in practice also requires that practitioners evaluate the *methodology* of their practice.

It is at this point that the cultivation of methodological antennae yields dividends. The general argument of the next few pages and much of the following chapter is that social workers' practice can be substantially enriched by an infusion of accommodated, translated and remodelled qualitative methods. Participant observation, qualitative interviews, developments in the application of focus groups, documentary sources and variations of life history methods all challenge ways in which social workers evaluate assessing and planning and, of course, all moments and phases of intervention. We consider participant observation, interviews and life history methods in this chapter and explore the potential of documents, focus groups and other opportunities for reflexive evaluating in the next chapter.

Participant observation

The use of observation methods has an established pedigree in social work. Ranging from the use of non-participatory observers in clinical settings and the observation of created social worlds within groupwork, through the utilisation of informal observation for assessment purposes in residential units, to the unplanned, informal, participatory observations within youth and community work, no social workers would deny that they use information gained from observing those with and for whom they practice. Yet having conceded as much, the impression lurks that observation remains marginal to social work practice. Planned observation tends to be non-participatory, and seems to be regarded as an enthusiasm or specialism. Participant observation appears more often than not to be an accident of the substance of social work. Just as sociology has sometimes been labelled the science of the interview, so social work can be called, without too much risk of misrepresentation, the profession of the interview. It is a stark paradox that an occupation committed to understanding and working with people should have restricted the avenues of understanding and action to so many variants of the interview.

The scope for participant observation as an agency of better action and understanding, and thus as a means of better evaluating in practice, is elastic. Practice in hospitals, residential units, youth and community work, penal institutions, direct work with children, family intervention and assessment, social work with groups, and evaluating in the context of individual caseloads all lend themselves to participant observation. New challenges and difficulties are posed by such practice applications, which we outline below. If participant observation is 'the most intimate and morally hazardous method of social research' (Lofland, 1971: 93), then much the same will apply to participant observation in social work practice. But it is the very sharpness and excitement of dilemmas around ethical issues, role relations, the reactivity of observing, the reality of gendered relations, record making and keeping, understanding, and the special stress that observing brings, that provide a major part of the pay-off for observation methods. The same dilemmas are, of course, present in slightly different guises with practice based on interviews. We are simply less aware of them by virtue - or vice - of over-familiarity.

Patricia Searight in her extensive self-evaluation of her own practice as a family therapist with children and young people from the ages of six to nineteen who had been diagnosed as having a behaviour disorder also explored a version of participating and evaluating (Searight, 1988). While she was not focusing solely on assessment and planning, her work will serve as a vignette to illustrate the potential of participant observation. In contrast to the context-stripping tendencies of the dominant mode of evaluation, she explored the impact on self-evaluation of the various contexts of her practice, in addition to the perspectives and symbolic meanings of clients, practitioners and the co-therapists with whom she worked. Her observation was mainly of direct therapy events, on the grounds that the evaluator needs to participate in the person's world of *meanings*, but not necessarily in the client's *environment*. These events included activities in homes and in the community, talking, playing cards and games, video watching, cooking, eating, listening to music, drawing and painting. She audio-taped all her sessions. Her perspectives changed during the sixteen months that she sustained her evaluation - changes that stemmed partly from the process of self-evaluating and in part from the outcomes. For example, her assumption had been that the content of practice would consist of client lives outside the practice situation, and that self-reflection would be a major part of the sessions. Neither of these assumptions was upheld.

She suggested several ways in which the model has utility for practitioners. It forced her to redefine her practice as including not only skills but also the contexts of practice. The achievement of change and recurring doubts and loss of self-esteem were both better understood by being placed in the perspective of contexts as well as direct practice. It 'helps the worker to move away from over-personalising practice in the sense of the worker's skills equalling practice' (p328). This in turn constrained the way she defined practice evaluation and criteria for effectiveness. She advocates

> a concept of practice effectiveness which is more than the successful use of skills by the worker, more than the appropriateness of actions by the worker, and more than the accomplishment of agreed upon goals...An evaluation of practice must include assessment and judgements of the interactions between clients and workers, according to each of the actors' perspectives (p326).

Evaluating in practice carried out on this scale is probably not feasible for most practitioners. Indeed, she found it impossible to find time to work through the mass of tape recorded sessions and events while working in that agency. This was partly a problem of scale but also one of role and perspective. She 'could not focus on data collection and be a full participant in practice evaluations simultaneously' (p312). Her final analysis of her self-evaluation could only be completed after she had left that practice setting and was working in another agency. She needed to reflect *on* action as well as reflect *in* action (Schon, 1983: 126).

There are two ways in which Searight's model might be changed to render it more feasible for day-to-day practice. First, she is surely right to conclude that 'it does not seem realistic to expect practitioners to conduct systematic self-evaluations of their practice' (335). A targeted evaluation is both more feasible and less likely to encounter evaluation-fatigue. Second, the isolation involved in carrying out extensive evaluating in practice poses additional problems when working in a team, a project or an agency where there is no culture of self-evaluation. An inbuilt mentor or consultant role, perhaps from a social science research base in higher education, will probably prove a helpful counterweight.

Issues of consent, access, trust, and observer roles do not figure strongly in Searight's account, but are part and parcel of participant observation. Social work with children is a part of practice where participant observation is possible, and where these issues occur in a distinct way (Shaw, 1996). Understanding the world of childhood pulls with both fascination and mystery. How many of us have delved into Iona and Peter Opie's books both to learn and to remember (eg Opie and Opie, 1959; 1969)? The problem with 'Kid Society' (the term is Glassner's) is their physical closeness and social distance. 'Our proximity to children may lead us to believe that we are closer to them than we really are - only differing in that...children are still growing up...and they are often wrong' (Fine and Sandstrom, 1988: 34). The value of participant observation is that we need to make these neighbours into strangers and by that route into peers if we are to get a sense of what it means to be a child, and be able to view the world 'through their hearts and minds' (p12). In doing so we will struggle to mine our own experience, and be challenged to breech our own well-constructed defences.

Perhaps the single most important decision that a practitioner will take in deciding to observe with children is the nature of the observer role. This may range from the detached observer - not unlike the conventional use of observation facilities in clinical practice - through the 'special friend' role adopted by Corsaro (1985) in his excellent study of children in a nursery school, to the active, fully participating 'least adult role' practised by Mandell (1988) in observing two pre-school centres. Mandell advocates suspending all adult-like characteristics except physical size, and taking a role which minimises social distance, suspends judgements on children's immaturities, engages in joint action with children, and risks being taken for a fool.

Observational studies of children have fallen into three kinds. There are those which find that children are more mature or capable than we expect, observations that deromanticise childhood and find they are more tendentious or rebellious, and finally those that shed light on how the secret process of education, or socialisation by peers, occurs. Fine and Sandstrom remark that 'we know of no study that has found that children are more 'childish' than we have given them credit for' (p72). The challenge for any social worker who chooses to observe with children is to 'capture the dynamics of children's interactions and to fit into children's interpretive acts without disturbing the flow' (Mandell, 1988: 464).

Ethical issues vary according to the age of the children or young people, and may be less of a problem with very young children because there are usually other adults who take on protective roles. The dilemma may arise when questions of adult responsibility in potentially harmful situations arise. For example, how should participating social workers respond to instances of racism or theft? The natural tendency of social workers may be to *challenge* the former and *observe* the latter. But social workers also need to observe the former, or they may run the risk of not *understanding* racist and sexist talk. Social workers may be called on to exercise 'reactive policing' by responding to complaints by one child against another, and other adults in the vicinity will inevitably act as if the observer is caring for their interests. But trust, informed consent, and the right of children to say 'no' remain central.

Interviewing and participant observation

If social work is the profession of the interview, then perhaps we can assume that social workers possess good enough skills in the use of interviewing as a channel for evaluating in practice. I am not persuaded. Interviews have been rightly developed as means of guaranteeing practice accountability, with the consequence that some styles of interviewing have become more common than others. Social work practitioners have perhaps been insufficiently sensitive to the essentially interactive nature of all interviews. Cicourel (1964) long ago argued that we need to see the interview empirically, as one variation of interaction in everyday life, and as an example of encounters with strangers. Rees has suggested that social work interviews can be viewed in a similar light (Rees, 1974). 'Bias' and distortion should be viewed as normal, commonsense responses, and it will prove impossible to have a standardised interview presentation. The social typification of interviewer roles varying between culture and class, the constant interaction tension as one person tries to penetrate the private world of another, and the advantages and disadvantages of rapport, must all be made part of social workers' awareness when evaluating the implications of relying on interviews in normal practice.

Interview styles developed for qualitative research purposes are equally marked by these interactional features, yet they are more likely to offer a sound framework for evaluating in practice. To pursue the example of social work practice with children, careful criticisms have been developed of the use of clinical interviews with children (Siegert, 1986; Bierman and Schwartz, 1986). These point to the inherent paradox of using interviews based on an asymmetrical adult-child relationship in order to learn about knowledge and behaviour that commonly arises in egalitarian relationships with friends and peers. Also, whereas social workers have traditionally been strong in understanding the impact of family dynamics, work which lends itself to social work application has been done which lays stress on understanding interviews with children as being filtered through the child's culture (Goode, 1986; Baker, 1983; Parker, 1984). Finally, the attention given to user involvement following the Care in the Community changes has helpfully pushed practitioners to consider appropriate ways of working with people on the receiving end of social work.   In exploring ways of giving a voice to people with learning disabilities, Pitcairn has provided much helpful, practical, and extremely well-founded advice on her experience of interviewing service users (Pitcairn, 1994; Atkinson, 1988).

What guidelines exist for social workers and service users who wish to adopt the best option for evaluating service provision? McKeganey looked with his colleagues at the process of decision making where professionals and clients meet to decide upon admission to homes for the elderly. They used both interviewing and participant observation methods, and drew out the costs and benefits of each method. Their conclusions will bear repeating and 'translate' fairly readily to other aspects of practice evaluating.

Interviews are better for collecting information about discrete cases. It is difficult to focus on cases through the use of observation because decisions about individuals occur across several contexts of place and time. Interviews can cover key decision points in a given case, and also offer the possibility of 'triangulating' different professionals' and service users' accounts. However, they do not resolve how to weigh different and conflicting accounts. Formal public components of practice are more readily identified through interviews.

If interviews yield a strong depiction of formal processes, 'one of the benefits of observational work is precisely the capacity to focus attention upon the informal aspects of professionals' decision making' (McKeganey, MacPherson and Hunter, 1988: 16). For example, routine decision making is often taken for granted. It may form part of people's tacit knowledge which they find hard to articulate. Observation may tap into these taken for granted practices and responses. Furthermore, Schutz made a telling criticism of positivist research which excludes motives and intentions, to the effect that it has no means of identifying decisions *not* to do something (Schutz, 1979). There is no easy solution to these problems in that both participant observation and interviewing may miss this element of intentionality.

Interviews present additional problems because they tend to recreate past decisions as if they were more rational than in fact they were. This is partly due to the inevitable problems of needing to rely on memory questions to reconstruct the past. The validity problems arising from memory questions have been insufficiently addressed by social workers. There are five main kinds of problems (Marsh, 1982). First, we tend to telescope past events, and are thus liable to overestimate the connection between events and situations. Second, we 'remember' by matching events to stereotypes. We have already discussed the process of reflective evaluating in practice in terms of testing those stereotypes. Third, memory is selective and unrepresentative. Fourth, we tend to underestimate socially un-desirable events and behaviours and overestimate socially desirable ones. What counts as socially desirable or undesirable will, of course, be shaped by cultural constraints, as was pointedly illustrated by Scott's work with mothers using a maternal and child health centre, described earlier in this chapter. Fifth, service users are often asked to recall matters such as housing conditions or marital status. These are not events as such but are aspects of ongoing situations (Marsh calls them 'situational variables'). Social workers may, as a result, be tempted to oversimplify cause and effect arguments. Cause and effect inferences need care for another reason. If one event or behaviour happens *before* another, it does not follow that the first has *caused* the second. Human beings 'have the capacity to anticipate future events and take account of them before they happen' (Marsh, 1982: 83).

Observational work can elicit the more chaotic nature of present decisions, but cannot learn directly about the past. Finally, in understanding the moral valuations that service users and practitioners accord to practice, subjective, moral and perhaps pejorative categories may be used in less-formal settings. Observation methods are more likely than interviews to reveal these user and practitioner judgements.

Life stories

An important element of social work practice involves 'taking histories', whether they be for assessment purposes, reports, or as part of clinical interventions. Evaluating in practice will be enriched by thinking afresh of practice as entailing an understanding of histories. The construction of life stories brings together the participatory aspect from observation methods and the interactive character of qualitative interviews. The use of various forms of life story methods has been a valuable area of interest in more recent social work practice. It has helped to enrich work with children through life stories, and its selective use through reminiscence work with older people has introduced to that field a welcome human touch. Our concern here is the re-orienting of that work to utilise its potential for evaluating in practice.

There are several contributory sources entering the stream of life history work. Within sociology the creative explosion of 1930s research in the Chicago School produced an exciting tradition of ethnography (Becker, 1970), marked by 'a horizontal and vertical reading of the biography and the social system; back and forth from biography to social system, and from social system to biography' (Bertaux, 1981, quoted by Clifford, 1994). Oral history work, developmental psychology and social gerontology have also influenced work in this field. More recent work within sociology has re-awakened interest in personal and life documents. One development of this kind that has potential application within social work is life course sociology (Morgan, 1985; Clapham, Means and Munro, 1993; Clifford, 1994).

> The essence of life course sociology is that it places change and development at the centre of the analysis of personal and family lives, and makes connections between 'family time', 'individual time', and 'historical time'
>
> (Clifford, 1994: 109).

Bowen's essay (1993) on the delights of learning to apply the life history method to school non-attenders conveys the commitment of a practitioner working at an innovatory means of understanding and action. He had about twelve weekly meetings with four people who had been in care and who had experienced education problems, but who were not known previously to him. After gaining their confidence he secured eight or nine hours of tape recorded conversation with each of them. Three of them - all, of course, with serious education problems - wrote autobiographies ranging from 5000 to 12,000 words. Bowen's impressive work is sufficient to demonstrate the considerable potential for applying life history work to assessing and planning, and to evaluating that work, particularly in circumstances where time is available and there is no crisis needing immediate drastic intervention. Martin has written helpfully and more generally on oral history in assessment and intervention (Martin, 1995).

Life course sociology has a range of possible applications. Unlike the life cycle approaches more familiar to social workers, life course analysis 'places change and development at the heart of the analysis and seeks to explore the inevitable temporal dimension of our lives and experiences' (Morgan, 1985: 177). Therefore it is not simply a technique to add to the social worker's armoury, but also a means of empowering the individuals and families with whom we work.

Clapham's description of the use of life course housing biographies with older people points to one area where reminiscence work can be re-directed and enhanced and can provide a basis for informed decision making in relation to housing and accommodation decisions by older people and their families. Clapham also stresses that the method has valuable predictive uses as a forward planning instrument. We

> need to see old age, and housing in old age, as stages in the life course which can only be understood by reference to previous experience and the attitudes and choices of people and the opportunities open to them during the whole life course
>
> (Clapham, Means and Munro, 1993: 133).

Housing biographies involve constructing a personal biography through in-depth qualitative interviews in order to understand how people got to their present housing situation. Strong emphasis is necessary on why certain options were chosen and especially why other options were rejected. The biography will include *individual* time, reflected, for example, in age and state of health; *family* time demonstrated in the stage of the family life cycle, and *historical* time as evidenced in the prevailing economic, social and political conditions (Morgan, 1985).

There are certain risks to be avoided if possible. For example, class, gender and ethnic differences do not disappear with old age. Also, choices must not be overemphasised at the expense of recognising constraints. This problem can arise 'particularly because of the "taken-for-granted" nature of many of the societal constraints which influence the way that people perceive the options open to them' (Clapham *et al*, 1993: 143).

Judgements will also need reaching regarding the 'validity' of life history accounts. General considerations of plausibility and the use of member evaluation methods of the kind discussed in the next chapter come into play. Clifford argues for a critical life history approach which draws together various strands of the methods outlined above, and offers an anti-oppressive method. He believes that life stories can be seen as *both* myth and history. The myth is valuable because of what it tells us about prevalent myths at that time, but he argues also that the account is 'real'. In the same way,

Burchardt concluded from her study of stepchildren's memories that 'reality is less tidy than myth. Time and again real personal experience breaks through, at times negating the myth, taking the story in unexpected directions, and finally giving its own substance to every life story' (Burchardt, 1990: 249).

We can reach a number of conclusions from this chapter regarding good evaluating in practice when setting the agenda for assessment and planning. It will be based on an understanding of competence that is not narrowly skills-based but which addresses the application of values and principles and is marked by a constant search for negative instances. Feminist evaluators will seek to institutionalise 'outsider within' ways of seeing when evaluating assessment and planning. Project development work will be marked by self-critical and informed claims making.

Evaluating assessment and planning will be characterised by a methodological alertness to the various possibilities of adapting qualitative research methods. These will include participant observation, a critical comparison and choice between qualitative interviews and observation methods, and the development of precedents found in life history and life course sociology. In the following chapter we will develop further opportunities for challenging agenda and methodologies within social work intervention processes.

8   Social work in action: evaluating the process of practice

'Well', says Howard...'it's a very interesting story'. 'The trouble is', says Flora, picking up her handbag, and feeling into its interior, 'I'm not sure it is. Isn't a story usually a tale with causes and motives? All I've told you is what happened.' 'Perhaps it's a very modern story,' says Howard, 'a chapter of accidents.'

Malcolm Bradbury ('*The History Man*')

In this chapter we explore themes, strategies and tactics for evaluating social work interventions.   The practitioner works 'in a forest of events and stories pointing inward and outward, and backward and forward.'   Stories given by service users and practitioners are marked by feelings, hopes, beliefs, environmental realities, the retention of the past and the fitting of the story into a future horizon whereby 'there is a sense of history even before there is a history' (Clandinin and Connelly, 1994: 417, 418).

We will pick up from earlier in the book the themes of personal narrative, participatory evaluation, self and practitioner evaluation, to illustrate how they permeate inquiry into the processes and actions of intervention. In the second half of this chapter we sketch additional examples of how qualitative methodology can be translated, remodelled and accommodated to the purposes of evaluating in practice.   We consider the relevance of documents for practice evaluation, advocate the utilisation of developments in focus group methods, and illustrate several reflexive review methods whereby practitioners and service users may get 'unstuck' in social work practice. In doing so we seek to rescue evaluating in practice from being 'culture-bound' (Rees, 1987), and avoid the risk of *post hoc* justification that sometimes characterises social workers' defence of practice decisions. The approach followed in this chapter is similar to the previous chapter. We first suggest ways in which evaluating in practice addresses the *agenda* of intervention processes, and will proceed from there to describe how it challenges the *methodology* of intervention.

The distinction between formative and summative evaluation has become part of the vocabulary of evaluation literature. Formative evaluation of social work practice inquires into the delivery and implementation of services - the process and story of social work in action - and considers how it might be improved. Summative evaluation addresses the impact of the intervention process, its outputs and outcomes. This chapter deals with formative evaluating in practice, while Chapter Nine covers summative evaluating in practice. In reality the distinction is not clearcut. Social work intervention cannot be separated from either assessment and planning or practice outcomes. Practice assessments and plans are not achieved by passive observers. To accomplish an assessment of what is really going on, a social worker will often need to be proactive and seek a response, so that 'intervention precedes or is simultaneous with diagnosis.' Not only so, but 'diagnostic efforts are themselves interventions of unknown consequences' (Schein, 1987: 29).

Just as intervention cannot be split from assessment, neither can it be sealed off from service outcomes. For example, in social group work changes in relations between group members may be viewed either as a means through which changes in the group members' lives outside the group can be accomplished, and therefore as part of an intervention process or as the end-goal of practice, and thus an outcome. Confusion between intervention and outcome is also produced by the realities of practice. This was illustrated when Humphrey and Pease (1992) asked probation officers about their effectiveness, and found that they were often answered in terms of service inputs such as number of pre-sentence reports (PSR's) completed or numbers of community sentence orders achieved, rather than in terms of outputs. They suggest that the reason for this may lie partly in probation officers' assumptions about the intrinsic worth of PSR's. If PSR's are seen as a good in themselves and this goodness is more or less taken for granted, then they will tend to be seen as 'virtual outputs'. In the accounts of social workers earlier in this book, we saw that beliefs about the complexity of practice, limited accountability and the influence of 'luck' in shaping the outcomes of practice all served to complicate the perceived relationship between practice and outcomes. For these reasons the distinction between formative and summative evaluating in practice is treated as a useful device but no more.

Personal, practitioner and participatory

Evaluating the process of practice has a three-pronged starting line. *First*, evaluating in practice involves crafting meaning out of the stories that people live and tell. Social workers are not interested in experience as such, but in experience bounded by social work questions and purposes. Social work practitioners are sometimes guilty of reductionism, whereby skills and techniques obscure experience. In saying this we do not intend to suggest the romantic notion that social workers may have direct access to the raw sensation of clients' lives, but rather that stories are the closest we can come to experience. Experience 'is the stories people live. People live stories, and in the telling of them reaffirm them, modify them and create new ones' (Clandinin and Connelly, 1994: 415). Therefore, 'there is a reflexive relationship between living a life story, telling a life, retelling a life story, and reliving a life story' (p418). Oral histories, plans, journals, photographs, family stories, letters, children's stories, and conversations are the personal texts for a shared narrative inquiry between practitioners and service users.

Second, evaluating the process of practice is practitioner evaluation. Indeed, much of the recent discussion of 'participatory' inquiry means precisely this, that professionals and managers who may traditionally rely entirely on outside 'experts' to evaluate for them, should be drawn in as participatory, practitioner-evaluators. In Peter Reason's words this is about transforming 'people who in orthodox research would be...subjects into co-researchers', on the grounds that 'we can only truly do research *with* persons if we engage with them *as* persons, as co-subjects and thus as co-researchers' (Reason, 1994a: 3, 10). Miller and Crabtree have advocated the application of qualitative methods to clinical research - a territory which has traditionally been the province of clinical trial methods based on 'control through rationality' (Miller and Crabtree, 1994: 342).

They identify three tasks which need to be addressed if qualitative practitioner evaluation is to flourish. First, an 'open space' needs creating that welcomes such approaches. For this to happen the questions must emerge from the practice experience outlined in Chapters Three and Four of this book, and the results must be directed to all practice participants. Second, social work participants, including those who work in research and higher education, must provide the tools necessary for discovering and testing practice stories and knowledge claims. Finally, ways must be identified and described whereby practice stories and knowledge can be shared. Qualitative evaluators no longer need to speak in language that seeks to justify their craft to an unsympathetic world. In line with our earlier comments in Chapter Six on the validity and plausibility of evaluating in practice, practice stories and knowledge can be shared if they are convincing in methodological, rhetorical and practice terms. *Methodologically*, the evaluating must tell the evaluators' relationship with 'informants' and also with the audience. Evaluating is *rhetorically* convincing if it 'assures the reader that the author has walked in their shoes' (Miller and Crabtree, 1994: 348). It is convincing in *practice* terms if it makes practice sense. 'Sense', that is, not in terms of conventionally received wisdom, but by being willing to stretch out our minds beyond the reach of the obvious.

Hilary Traylen's co-operative inquiry project with health visitors illustrates the potential of this kind of practitioner evaluation, in ways which could readily be applied to small peer groups of social work colleagues (Traylen, 1994). Five health visitors met with Traylen approximately monthly over about nine months, to address issues of hidden agendas in their practice which were not revealed when they visited families. They decided to work on how they might best confront families. Over several months they worked through cycles of hearing each others' methods, agreeing and refining inquiry methods to be adopted by the health visitors in their visits and returning to action. The establishment of a co-operative inquiry group working through cycles of inquiry is the central feature of the co-operative inquiry method, which owes something to the traditions of action research outlined in Chapter Two. The practitioners were heavily preoccupied with action rather than the research process over the early months and found it took some time to achieve the best balance between action and reflection. However, reflection revealed the centrality of story telling methods and the empowering impact of each cycle of inquiry.

A different tradition of self-evaluation by practitioners has developed rather patchily in voluntary organisations, federal community development agencies, and self-help groups (Meadows and Turkie, 1988; Robb and Hasen 1991; Adams, 1990; Hawtin, Hughes, Percy-Smith and Forman, 1994).   The growth of the performance culture during the 1980s prompted some voluntary agencies to set their own agenda for evaluation.   Although most voluntary organisations do not have many resources to use for the evaluation process, helpful accounts are available for agencies to use.   Meadows and Turkie, for instance, point to the need to clarify who the 'self' is in self-evaluation.   They point out that evaluation should be seen as a means of developing and not just reviewing the organisation, and offer a sound checklist of issues to address.   Most practitioners in this field accept the shared involvement of outside experts, if only as a means of securing credibility.

The *third* prong is that evaluating practice process must be participatory in the richer sense of involving the service user.   Telling stories has the potential to be empowering insofar as participants are given a voice.   As first steps to achieving this social workers must insert themselves in the other's story as a way of coming to know that story.   Indeed, both practitioner and service user need to enjoy the degree of mutual respect in which they both feel they have a voice to tell their stories.

Whitmore's account of an evaluation of a pre-natal programme for single expectant mothers illustrates how this may sometimes be achieved through feminist participatory evaluation.   The evaluation was carried out over several months by four women who had themselves been through the programme, with Whitmore as consultant to the project.   There were tensions in the group.   One member left, and there were communication failures.   One participant protested to the consultant that

> Our world is different from yours.   The fear is that people always want to humiliate you, put you down (for being on welfare)...We have a different lifestyle from you.   We just don't trust people the way you do.
>
> (Whitmore, 1994: 92).

But the strength of their final achievement, leading also to presentations to the project advisory group, a conference, and a university class, is evidence that participatory evaluation with oppressed groups is not only political rhetoric.   The limitations of this kind of study arise from the recognition of recent feminist analysis that there is no single woman's experience which may be shared across boundaries of class, race, education and language.   Whitmore concluded that she could never entirely share the worlds of the women with whom she worked. 'My small words were often their big words. What I assumed was "normal talk", they saw as "professor words".' Martin arrived at similar conclusions from her own feminist participative research. She was unable to overcome the mystique associated in the minds of participants with research, or the relationship of 'anti-dialogue' created by the cultural invasion of the researched by the researcher. She reasons that feminist participative research 'places unrealistic expectations on the extent to which the researched can become involved in the research process', and concludes that 'even when problems are of a major concern to people (the researched) they have work and private lives which usually take priority, whereas research IS work for the researcher' (Martin, 1994: 142).

Participatory evaluating in practice also emphasises the way in which relations between participants are gendered. We noted this in passing in the previous chapter when advocating the development of participatory observation methods for evaluating assessment and planning. Service users will have gendered expectations regarding both within-gender and cross-gender relations with practitioners. Reflecting on participatory research in therapeutic communities, in an adolescent drugs unit and in home help services, McKeganey and Bloor concluded that there are two aspects of gendered relations that are likely to be given insufficient recognition. First, although cultural blindness to same sex relations made access to males easier for them as male researchers, the activities and conversations of within-gender relations were still markedly gendered. Second, in cross-gender relations sexual interpretations may be made when the researcher is not aware.

> In everyday life there is recurrent slippage between gendered relationships and relationships with a sexual component. Many everyday asexual relationships frequently become problematic or ambiguous for one or both participants, with one party considering a possible sexual interpretation of an utterance or action of another
>
> (McKeganey and Bloor, 1991 :209).

Social work evaluating of the process of practice must be participatory, practitioner-led, and personal. If it is to be personal, what is the relationship between personal narrative and the records and documents that provide the every-day bridge between practice and the agency?

Personal texts and practice texts

The relationship between service users' personal experience, stories and texts, and social workers' restorying of that experience in their informal narratives of client work, case records, and inter-agency reports, presents one of the most difficult problems for social work practice in general and for evaluating social work process in particular. It is however, rarely considered in the literature on practice and evaluation. The brief debate here builds on our discussion of life histories in Chapter Seven. Full reflection on the issues is beyond our scope, and the beginnings of a fuller groundwork can be found in the sources cited here and in the previous chapter.

Personal texts may, of course, be either oral or written. They may have been storied or restoried for a social work audience, although most personal service user texts have a life in themselves without influence by the social worker. Practice texts, by virtue of their audience, are usually written. Figure 8.1 outlines a basic categorisation for personal and practice texts, grouped according to the usual degree of access that may be had to those texts (Scott, 1990). The dimension of 'access' refers to the availability of documents to people other than their authors. Documents subject to 'closed' access are those which are available only to a limited circle of eligible insiders. 'Restricted' documents are accessible on an *ad* hoc basis under specified conditions to those outsiders who are able to secure the permission of the insiders. 'Archival' access exists where the documents have been lodged in a place of storage which is open to all outsiders subject only to fairly minimal administrative procedures. Finally, 'published' documents are the most open of all, being printed for public circulation. The distinctions of access and of personal/practice should not be used as a reason to fix texts in reified categories. Which cell an example fits into will vary according to power, motive, intention, purpose and the results of negotiation. To ignore this would simply mirror the tendency for welfare records to become institutionalised, rigid and inflexible, whereby social categories change but record categories become ingrained.

Access	Personal	Practice
Closed	Client diaries Personal correspondence	Agency case records 'Personal' case records Housing records
Restricted	Family stories Client life stories written for social worker Photo collections and other personal/ family artefacts	Service contracts Case committee minutes Equal opportunities data Reports to other agencies
Archive	Family correspondence archive Photographic records	Voluntary society archive Performance indicator reports Community profiles Funding bids
Published	Published client accounts of social work experience	Annual agency reports School/hospital 'league tables' Census reports

Figure 8.1   Social work texts

In distinguishing different personal texts that will be relevant to practitioner, participatory and personal evaluating, I will follow closely the outline in Clandinin and Connelly's incisive review of personal experience methods in qualitative research, together with their earlier research work carried out in school settings (Clandinin and Connelly, 1994; Connelly and Clandinin, 1990). They distinguish between annals and chronicles. Annals can be envisaged as a 'line' which schematises an individual's life divided into moments or segments by events, places, years or significant memories. This allow a sense of the whole, including highs and lows, and the rhythms they construct around their life cycle. Chronicles are an elaboration of a single point in the annal. Both together are 'a way to scaffold their oral histories' (1994: 420), and re-collect their experiences. They are also a way to begin to hear a person's family stories. These family stories are handed down across generations about family members and events. Through them people learn self-identity, both internally and in the relation of the family to the world. It is the atypicality and on occasion impoverishment of family stories that mark many people with whom practitioners work. Photographs, correspondence, trinkets and other artefacts mark times, events and persons around which stories are constructed and reconstructed, often by women to children.

Journals provide a way of giving accounts of experience. Clandinin and Connelly quote a delightful analogy to the effect that journal entries were to one woman like tiny children's sweets which are so small that separately they are not worth eating, but which together provide a pattern of enjoyment. Children and adolescents often keep journals of their thoughts, activities and stories. Most of these remain private, and it is usually only the accident of history that brings to public view the childhood writings of an Anna Frank or the Bronte children. Childhood memories of those who come within the sphere of influence of social workers are more often emotions recollected in the relative tranquillity of older years (eg Courtney, 1989). But it is likely that some children and young people with whom practitioners work keep journals as attempts to make sense of their experiences - 'capturing fragments of experience in attempts to sort themselves out' (1994: 421). Adults speaking of their experiences as a child raise special difficulties for the hearer. Who is speaking?

> Is it the adult interpreting the childhood experience, in which case it is the adult speaking. Or is it the adult expressing the child's story as the child would have told the experience, in which case it is the child speaking
> (1994: 424).

The texts of personal experience disclose the scene and plot, the dimensions of place and time. Plot, meaning and interpretation are far from straightforward, especially as practitioner and service user seek to understand meaning when they are evaluating practice. Today's meanings may become items in tomorrow's chronicle of events, as the participants change their understandings. We have tried to make clear our conviction that social workers operate at a point too far removed from the experience and stories of those with whom they work.

There are ethical considerations that need careful guarding. 'Personal experience methods are relationship methods' (1994: 425), and the 'evaluation contract' will usually need making explicit. The ordinary contract-in-use between social workers and clients is likely to run along the lines that the client receives help, advice, or punishment in the community in relation to an issue which the social worker or others define as a problem for the client and probably for others. In return the client accepts the role and pays any costs in terms of time, expenses, lost opportunities or stigma. The practitioner will give time, skills, a filter to resources and so on, within (uncertain) standards about confidentiality. The terms of a contract for participatory, practitioner, personal evaluating in practice will need time consuming negotiation. It was a feature of the instances of evaluating cited earlier in this chapter (Traylen, 1994; Whitmore, 1994) that the evaluating contract took some time to be achieved. Ethical issues are also raised by the fact that as we encourage service users to tell their stories, we become characters in those stories, and thus change those stories. This can be positive, and be one way of helping someone to get 'unstuck' in their work on a problem, but it also carries risks and re-emphasises that evaluating must be done with care and not as 'a raid on mislaid identities' (Dannie Abse's phrase, from his poem *Return to Cardiff*, cf Stacey, 1988).

Practice texts and documents may seem altogether more familiar territory to social workers when compared with personal texts. Yet the boundary is not at all watertight, and the assumption we have made in this discussion is that documents of practice organisations are only one instance of documents of life. The permeability of this boundary is immediately evident, for example, when we realise that social workers have on occasion been given (helpful) advice to keep *personal* notebooks consisting of working notes about significant data, inferences and provisional analyses of practice (Siporin, 1975). When assessing the value of practice texts as an ingredient of evaluating in practice, social workers need a framework which recognises their socially constructed nature yet allows space for such texts to throw light on practice.

Practice texts can be assessed against four criteria (Scott, 1990). Are they authentic? In other words, is a text genuine as to its authorship and origin? Second, are they credible? Credibility includes the two aspects of accuracy and sincerity. Third, is the evidence typical of its kind? This is the test of representativeness. Finally, what does the text mean? Is the meaning clear and comprehensible?

Authenticity is not usually a problem for social workers in that they are not normally working with historical texts but with the original. The continued growth in the use of information technology increasingly removes some of the threats of copy error. The test of *credibility* is a more difficult one for social work practice texts to satisfy. The accuracy and 'sincerity' of records both come under threat. The test of sincerity is whether the authors believed what they recorded. Social workers routinely select what they record in the light of the anticipated audience. Scott suggests that the best filter of sincerity is to ask what material interest the author had in the audience reaction to the record. For example, reports to courts may often function as 'sad tales' which emphasise determinist, and hence by inference relatively 'excusable', interpretations of behaviour. This brings us immediately up against the character of records as socially produced texts. Hall's illuminating work on the way in which social work duty teams 'produce' clients (1979) demonstrated that the social production of practice texts begins with the baseline decision of whether a citizen becomes categorised as a client.

Credibility defined as *accuracy* is often jeopardised for social workers by the fact that their records are often not eye witness accounts. The main partial exceptions to this are residential settings, and some group work and family therapy work. Part of the argument in the last chapter regarding the absence of observation methods in social work was an argument about credibility. The point needs more carefully stating. Practice texts are usually not eye witness accounts of *behaviour*, although they may more often be eye witness accounts of *attitudes* and perhaps *beliefs*. However, even in these cases written practice texts often suffer credibility threats arising from the lapse of time between practice and 'writing up' that practice. We should not conclude from this that written accounts will always be superior to spoken, oral texts. For example, Sainsbury discovered that client memories of some aspects of social work practice were fuller and more accurate than practitioner records of the same event

(Sainsbury, 1975). It is possible that in a subculture where writing is not the customary means of preserving evidence and memories, oral accounts may be more accurate. A reading of the work on oral history would illumine and enrich social work practice in this regard (eg Thompson, 1978; Samuel and Thompson, 1990).

The selectivity that threatens the credibility of a text also risks jeopardising its *representativeness*. For example, records of inquiries to a social services duty team are likely to be selective and therefore not representative of all the inquiries that are made. But selectivity is not only about selective *deposit*, but also about selective *survival* and *decay* (Webb *et al*, 1966). It is possible that the growing use of information technology will pose new problems of this kind. For instance, will machine stored data on hard disk be systematically transferred to new machines as one generation of hardware is relatively quickly replaced by another? Will back-up copies be routinely created and stored? A different problem of repre-sentativeness arises from the widely varying extent to which access to texts is possible (Figure 8.1). If texts vary in availability, the texts we can *use* will be unrepresentative, even if the texts from which they are taken are entirely representative. We referred earlier to personal texts created by service users especially for practice purposes. It goes without saying that such texts will almost certainly be unrepresentative of unsolicited personal texts, although it would be unwise to exaggerate the difference, given the nature of all personal texts as storied lives.

The most extensive threat to the potential of practice texts for evaluating revolves around decisions about the *meaning* of those texts. Scott is commenting on medical records but his strictures apply with similar force to some social work records.

> The clinical folder is elliptical and vague, resting on a vast body of taken-for-granted assumptions, and its therapeutic meaning can only be grasped by participants who understand the situation in which it was produced. The record is constructed so as to allow...staff to reconstruct the therapy and so legitimate their action
>
> (Scott, 1990: 124).

Practitioners and managers will read practice records with very different agenda. Practitioners will see them as records of service, which 'document' the contractual relationship between social worker and client. The text will therefore be viewed as being about work accomplished through the relationship between them and whether obligations have been met. Managers and administrators are likely to view the same record as an 'actuarial' record (p124), and part of a system of supervision and monitoring which will provide an adequate basis for recording accountability to outside audiences. Records which may be regarded as 'poor' by administrators may begin to make sense when seen as the ingredients for a possible service contract. The consequent tension was neatly captured some years ago by Pearson (1975) when making his case that violations of professional values have a systematic and patterned character arising from the rough and tumble of the social worker's everyday practice. For example, professional codes claim that the client has a right to expect that communications should have confidential status. Yet 'the client's communications to officials of a public service, involving as they do matters of public money, and in the last analysis public order, have the character of public knowledge' (p53). Professional social work values also claim that the client has the right not to be judged by the social worker, yet 'the client's actions, by their nature problematic to "consensus", are judged' (p53).

An awareness of the socially produced nature of practice texts can help the practitioner to counter these effects and deal with records critically but also as resources of information for evaluating practice. Scott concludes that 'we must recognise three aspects of the meaning of a text - three "moments" in the movement of the text from author to audience' (p134). We must distinguish the meaning the author *intended* to produce and the *received* content, or the meaning constructed by the audience. We should not assume that there is just one intended or received meaning. Texts typically have multiple meanings. But there is also a third meaning of the text, as constructed by readers who were not members of the original intended audience. For example, a social worker may intend a community care contract to be a means of empowering service users. A line manager may see the same document as a more or less adequate protection of agency accountability. A subsequent reader may interpret it as reinforcing or challenging conventional gender roles. Texts may have meanings beyond their intentions. But as soon as a third party reads a text to interpret its meaning, she or he becomes part of its audience.

We have treated personal and practice texts as part of a single whole, and believe that this provides the basis for a richer and broader appreciation of such texts as part of practice evaluation.

Focus groups

Evaluations of social group work have paid too little attention to group process. A review of fifty-four studies focused entirely on group outcome evaluations, and also found that thirty-seven of these studies were of groups using cognitive-behaviour methods (Tolman and Molidor, 1994). These studies revealed no evidence of interest in evaluating in practice skills, and there has been very little attention to self-evaluation within the wider group care field (but see Collett and Hook, 1988-89).

One of the most promising developments in applying qualitative and participatory evaluation through groups has come through work on focus groups (Stewart and Shamdasani, 1990; Morgan, 1988; Morgan, 1993; Kreuger, 1994; Kitzinger, 1994). Focus groups originate from the unexpected quarter of market research, but also draw stimulus from the work of the American sociologist Robert Merton on focused interviews. They take the form of group discussions organised to explore a specific set of issues. 'The group is *focused* in the sense that it involves some kind of collective activity - such as viewing a film, evaluating a single health education message or simply debating a particular set of questions' (Kitzinger, 1994: 159). The planning and design of focus groups hinges mainly on decisions about the role of the group moderator, the development of the group agenda, the balance of openness and pre-structuring ('setting the agenda without setting the agenda' as Zeller describes it [Zeller, 1993]), recruitment methods, and decisions about group composition. Current best practice is to work with homogenous groups. 'Holding separate sessions with homogenous but contrasting groups is believed to produce information in greater depth than would be the case with heterogeneous groups' (Knodel, 1993: 40).

Focus groups have three particular advantages. First, the group interaction is itself the data - 'the interaction is the method' (Jarrett, 1993: 198). Kitzinger says in summary that the method 'enables the researcher to examine people's different perspectives as they operate within a social network and to explore how accounts are constructed, expressed, censored, opposed and changed through social interaction' (1994: 159). Second, focus groups are a form of participatory evaluation. They are valuable when there is a power differential between participants and decision makers, and hence have considerable potential for application within social work. Finally, they introduce a valuable approach to learning the extent of consensus on a particular issue. 'The co-participants act as co-researchers taking the research into new and often unexpected directions and engaging with each other in ways which are both complementary...and argumentative' (Kitzinger, 1994: 166).

The majority of writers in this field have opposed the application of focus groups to anything other than research or formal evaluation purposes. In my view this is an unhelpful generalisation. Focus groups have a particular contribution to make to evaluating in practice, which extends across assessment, planning, intervention and outcomes. Exercises in problem setting, project development, anti-discriminatory practice, addressing work that has become 'stuck', consumer feedback exercises, and working with sensitive topics, are all ways in which focus groups have something to offer to day-to-day practice evaluating.

Applications of the method to problem setting is illustrated in work in progress by Bloor and Shaw on estimating numbers of rough sleepers. Groups of homelessness experts met over two occasions to resolve the degree of consensus and disagreement regarding definitions of rough sleeping. Group members were presented with a brief agenda of questions, and a set of hypothetical cases, which they used to make explicit the underlying dimensions in their working definitions of rough sleeping. The groups were moderated by outside researchers and the discussions audio-taped.

Problem setting is often a central feature of early work in project development. 'Social research has not done well in reaching people who are isolated by the daily, exhausting struggles for survival, services and dignity' (Plaut, Landis and Trevor, 1993: 216). Plaut's account of the use of focus groups for community mobilisation among poor, white, politically conservative, rural communities illustrates how the method can lead to empowerment. Working as part of a larger project for community oriented primary health care, Plaut and colleagues organised extensive focus group work around small, subjectively identified, communities. Groups were asked to identify community health problems. A range of projects was initiated following the focus groups, and the groups became not only a source of data but 'a process for resident involvement in and legitimation of the project and its interventions' (p206). They conclude that the focus group is useful, not only as a research instrument 'but as a means whereby a community can recognise its needs within the framework of its own language and contexts, and mobilise accordingly' (p216-7). A variant of focus groups is also illustrated by Bond's account of a day's programme for three ten-year-old short- term foster girls, in which their views were sought about a family centre. A group discussion format was set up. Dressing up, food, painting, cooking, poster preparation, photography and a presentation were used in an innovative attempt to learn user views from children. It was a carefully planned initiative and exemplifies a potential for focus group work which falls well within the resources of most residential and day care settings (Bond, 1990-91).

The potential for empowering participants, and hence for anti-discriminatory evaluating, is also illustrated in Jarrett's work with black women at risk of long term poverty, and outside traditional family patterns. She observes that so far 'little attention has been given to focus group interviewing with low income and/or ethnic and racial minorities' (Jarrett, 1993: 200). She adopted imaginative recruitment methods through personal visits to sites in the American Head Start programme. She encountered some difficulties, similar to the issues that we mentioned earlier in this chapter in our discussion of feminist participatory evaluation. However, the groups produced evidence of a wide range and diversity, rapport seemed to be achieved, and viewpoints were examined intensively. Even when audience effect was evident, and group members performed for each other, the women in their groups 'themselves distinguished between performance-oriented accounts and serious talk' (p195). Butler and Williamson reached a similar conclusion in their group interviews with children. In understanding the purpose of humour they describe how some children display 'serious listening inside a funny shell' (Butler and Williamson, 1994: 46). Kitzinger's account of a programme using focus groups dealing with the effect of media messages about AIDS also illustrates the utilisation of the approach with socially marginalised groups.

Further potential applications could be developed, such as work with practitioners or service users when practice has become 'stuck', or consumer feedback as a development of the panel projects already used in some places with service users in the community care field. Kitzinger concludes that focus groups 'may be particularly effective when (they) draw together people who have previously been unable to share their experiences or who are physically isolated from one another, such as those caring for elderly relatives' (p169). Zeller's use of focus groups to learn about sexual decision making by young people suggests possible applications of the method to evaluating practice with sensitive problems (Zeller, 1993).

Despite the promise of this method for social work, focus groups should be used within their limitations. There is little or no research evidence on the relative benefits of focus groups over against interview methods (though see Kitzinger), and there are situations where focus groups probably should not be used. They should not be used if the practitioner's intention is to improve participants' communication or group skills. More generally, they should not be adopted for therapeutic purpose, or when the main purpose is to secure immediate action. If information, understanding or explanation are not central to the group's agenda, then other methods of intervention should be used. There are other practical constraints on focus group work. If personal views cannot readily be expressed in such a context or if breaches of confidentiality are likely to be a problem, then the method should not be used. When group members know each other particularly well, focus groups are also ill-advised. Finally, bearing in mind the benefits of homogeneous group membership, it is not advisable to run focus groups comprising both service users and social workers who hold case accountability for participants.

Reflexive evaluating of practice process

During the course of the last two chapters we have argued for the imaginative colonising of qualitative methods for evaluating social work assessments, plans and interventions. We have reviewed the potential of participant observation, qualitative interviews, life history methods, practice and personal texts and focus groups. Each of these strategies can be used to support a reflexive, falsifying, participatory and practitioner-led evaluating in practice. We will underscore the reflexive dimension of these strategies in the final paragraphs of this chapter through a brief outline of the potential of planned service user comment on practitioner evaluatings, the use of simulated clients, and the utility of detailed reviews of the practitioner's own experience of the practice issue.

Deep and long-lived familiarity with the culture of social work has the potential effect of dulling the practitioner's powers of observation. McCracken is discussing the use of long, qualitative interviews in social research, but his plea for detailed preliminary review of personal experience suggests a way of drawing on practitioners' intimate acquaintance with many of the issues that preoccupy service users. Such a 'cultural review' calls for minute examination.

> The investigator must inventory and examine the associations, incidents and assumptions that surround the topic in his or her mind...The object is to draw out of one's own experience the systematic properties of the topic
> (McCracken, 1988: 32).

In an application of this approach to the social meaning of 'free time' for carers of people with severe learning disabilities, Julia Shearn made the following list of 'associations, incidents and assumptions':

My definition of 'free time':

How I view 'free time' compared with 'working time'

My uses of free time

My choices regarding use of free time

What I plan, do not plan, and why

Infringements on my free time

My feelings when plans for free time are changed

My reactions when I have free time unexpectedly created

Times when I am unable to plan

Times when I have appointments during free time

This list illustrates the categories that would provide the basis for brief paragraphs of notes commenting on each item, and provides the basis for a reflexive accounting of free time. Evaluating practice in such a manner allows the conscious integration of personal and practice texts.

Reflexive elaboration of evaluating in practice can be taken a step further by inviting the service user to comment on the practitioner's views. A closely similar activity, usually described as 'member validation', has been carried out by some qualitative researchers

(Bloor, 1983; Emerson and Pollner, 1988). For example, Bloor describes member validation exercises with tonsillectomy consultants whose consultation decisions he had observed and analysed, and with staff of a therapeutic community where he had studied the relationship between the informal patient culture and the therapy programme (Bloor, 1983). There are several difficulties with this method that social workers will need to take into account. For example, commitment and motivation to collaborate in a fairly demanding exercise will need cultivating. In addition, the interview setting can lead to a pressure for consensus. 'An interview is a species of conversation and, as such, it follows the rules of polite conversation in which open disagreement is minimised' (Bloor, 1983: 162). The method also tends to assume that service users' views are fixed, whereas, as with the consumer studies of practice described in Chapter Four, consumer views may be contingent and provisional. But while consumer feedback cannot be treated as a test of the validity of the practitioner's understanding, these reasons are not sufficient to explain the disregard of member validation as an opportunity for reflexive work with service users. For example, it 'has not been used as often as perhaps one might expect in feminist research' (Olesen, 1994: 166).

Mutual reflexivity of this kind sometimes needs 'empirical fishing lines' (Graham Swift). Those who evaluate the process of practice come face to face with the invisibility of practice. How may we learn the ways in which social workers practice? How would different social workers deal with the same case? The methods we have discussed hitherto do not directly address this problem. A promising innovatory method has, however, been used by Wasoff and Dobash in their study of how a specific piece of law reform was incorporated into the practice of solicitors (Wasoff and Dobash, 1992; Wasoff and Dobash, 1996). The use of simulated clients in 'natural' settings allowed them to identify practice variations with some confidence that they could be ascribed to differences between lawyers and were not artefacts of different cases.

Suppose changes are introduced in the legislation and practice standards governing probation officers' work with people serving sentences in the community. Evaluators using simulated clients would prepare perhaps three detailed case histories designed to test the legal and practice issues under consideration. A researcher or evaluator takes on the role of the client in the case history. The probation officer interviews the 'client' within the 'natural' setting of a probation office. The interview is repeated by other probation officers, but using the same case history. Control over what is selected from the scenario is handed over to the probation officer.

The method is a development of role play methods, and yet it is quite different. Role play has been used almost entirely within training courses, and much less so in practice. Also role play has been used for skill development and not for practice understanding and evaluation. The administration of the exercise is also very different from role playing, in that the scenario is much more detailed, and the 'client' is the only one who is in a role. The probation officer or social worker is playing it as a real social worker, and the setting is not constructed. The use of simulated clients has several things going for it. First, social workers are familiar with the 'family' of methods from which it is drawn. Second, other methods are not always feasible for practical or ethical reasons. Simulated clients overcome the ethical problems of seeking the co-operation of genuine clients. Above all, thirdly, it makes practice visible. It will be clear from the brief description that the method could not be a tool for evaluating particular cases, but would focus on specific *kinds* of practice. The main value of the method is as a potential focus on practice development. When significant changes are being intro-duced that need to be evaluated, or when an agency or individual practitioner feels 'stuck' with this or that kind of problem, then the use of simulated clients offers a promising means of evaluating. The method needs some additional resourcing to prepare the case material, perhaps to act the role of clients, and to reflect on the quite detailed material that results from transcriptions of the interviews. The potential practice evaluation uses of this method are hinted at by Wasoff and Dobash, who conclude that the 'simulated client' may provide an additional research method for those studying professional/client relationships and interactions. It may also be extended to the study of elite groups in social work (for example, decision making at senior management levels), and to the study of the implementation of policy and professional discretion.

Good practice evaluating social work in action

We have seen over the course of the last two chapters that good evaluating in practice will entail the imaginative colonising of qualitative methods. Practitioner evaluating will draw on different strands of self-evaluation methods, and participatory evaluation will find ways of giving a voice to participant service users. Evaluating in practice will be enriched by an active recognition that personal and practice texts are both part of a wider category of life documents and texts. Personal texts disclose the dimensions of time and place which are part of the fabric with which good evaluating practice is 'made'. Practitioners will evaluate practice texts especially against standards of credibility, representativeness and meaning.

Focus groups have the potential for innovative application to evaluating problem setting, project development, community empowerment, anti-discriminatory practice, consumer feedback exercises, and work that has become 'stuck'. Finally, we have argued that reflexive evaluating in practice will include 'cultural reviews' of categories, planned service user feedback on evaluation, and the use of simulated clients in natural settings for purposes of practice development, and for reviewing areas of practice where progress has become intractable.

In Chapter Nine we will turn our attention from assessment, planning and process to evaluating outcomes in practice.

9   The end game: evaluating outcomes

In the dime stores and bus stations,
People talk of situations,
Read books, repeat quotations,
Draw conclusions on the wall.
Some speak of the future,
My love she speaks softly,
She knows there's no success like failure
And that failure's no success at all

Bob Dylan *('Love Minus Zero/No Limit')*

If somebody asked me, 'Do social workers in my team evaluate?', I think I'd have to reply 'Yes'...But maybe it's not evaluation in the terms other people would think of it, in terms of, sort of, **evidence,** or **proof** that things have certain outcomes.

Social worker

Social work works. A revival of confidence in the ability of social workers and probation officers to deliver effective interventions, and in the capacity of research to measure the outcomes of those interventions in a manner relevant to the enhancement of good quality practice, is persistently tugging at the coat tails of practitioners. If this confidence were to prove well founded, social work would be in a strong position. Able to satisfy the call of funders for accountable practice, the occupation would also be in a position to claim technical competence and, in turn, professional autonomy.

We will review this important assertion that social work is able to deliver an empirical practice that works, through a consideration of two of the most careful and widely held forms in which it is made. First, we will reflect on the debate within the Probation Service about the effectiveness of treatment strategies aimed at the rehabilitation of offenders. Were the negative conclusions drawn from research evaluations of probation practice in the 1960s and 1970s born of a premature mixture of inaccuracy and pessimism? Second, we will explore the widely supported claims for the benefits of the form of practitioner research represented by single-system designs. We will weigh the contribution that the empirical practice movement has so far made to evaluating in practice, and set alongside this the good practice prescriptions that follow from studies of service user satisfaction.

Unlike assessing, planning and intervening, service outcomes are not a phase within the social work process, but a 'product', either planned or unintended. They are associated with endings, whether of success, failure or ambiguity. As such they involve disengaging, giving a decent burial (the phrase is Peter Baldock's), conserving beneficial results, conducting various administrative tasks, evaluating the process and task achievements of the service users and private and public aspects of self evaluation (Henderson and Thomas, 1980). Yet while associated with endings, outcomes are in no way synonymous with closure. At the risk of repetition, it should be emphasised that distinctions between assessment, planning, intervention and outcomes are in large part heuristic devices which enable us to view aspects of practice from different perspectives. The consequences of practice, intended or otherwise, beneficial or harmful, are frequently idiosyncratic, in that they occur gradually, cyclically or separately in time from the period of intervention. The accounts of practitioners with which we started the argument of this book display a sensitivity to the complexity of these outcomes and consequences.

'Empirical fishing lines'

The integration of practice and research to form empirically based practice, achieved by a twin commitment to measuring and empiricism, represents the goal and strategy of achieving a practice that works. American academics and practitioner-researchers have led the way, from the early work of Scott Briar and Ed Thomas, through Bloom, Fischer, Hudson and Tripodi, to the more recent contributions of Blythe and in particular the writing of Bruce Thyer and the *Research on Social Work Practice* journal which he edits. Robert Ross in Canada, and Jim McGuire and Brian Sheldon in Britain have enriched this tradition.

Four planks exist in the argument for empirical practice. *First*, evidence has been produced in support of the case that some social work intervention has achieved a demonstrable effectiveness. *Second*, a cluster of intervention strategies organised around cognitive and behavioural methods is put forward as the exemplar of good practice on which this effectiveness has been based. Linked to this model of intervention is the *third* argument that the key to the integration of research and practice 'lies in the conception of the measurement process' (Blythe and Tripodi, 1989: 14; Blythe, Tripodi and Briar, 1995). *Finally*, a number of attempts have been made to widen the diffusion and implementation of empirical practice models within social work courses, and by means of monitored clinical trials and more substantial research programmes. Notwithstanding this, the meagre degree to which empirical models have become part of the staple fare of practice is a cause of lament to advocates of these models.

The apparent success of social work is sometimes explained as an artefact of a premature rejection of treatment interventions in the early 1970s. On this view social work was not shown to be inadequate but was inadequately measured. The argument from meta-analyses outlined later in this chapter is in part along these lines. However, the research-based claims for positive outcomes are more commonly explained in terms of better practice and conceptually and methodologically rigorous evaluation methods. The basic prescription for practitioners is believed to be,

- focus on the behaviour that needs targeting,
- have a clear problem definition,
- state and agree clear and structured objectives,
- adopt cognitive and behavioural treatment approaches,
- ensure that the planned intervention is delivered with technical 'integrity' (ie that the planned service is actually delivered), and
- maintain a strongly change-focused intervention.

Walter Hudson, for example, insists that 'if some form of change is not created, it is not possible to speak rationally about service effectiveness.' He argues that the basic strategy for empirical practice is simple and also that the philosophical problems of positivism alleged by critics are 'far more trivial than some would have us believe' (Hudson, 1988: 60, 63). The development of measurement technologies stems from the enthusiasm shown by protagonists of quantitative, positivistic approaches to research (eg Thyer, 1993). The case put forward is not simply that quantitative approaches are *better* than qualitative ones, but rather that quantitative approaches stand for *all* evaluation and that 'qualitative data...can readily be transformed to measurement scales' (Blythe and Tripodi, 1989: 19). Thyer has thrown out an uncompromising challenge to advocates of qualitative evaluation.

> Social work practitioner-researchers look in vain for qualitative research studies which have clearly demonstrated the effectiveness of social work intervention in solving problems of social importance
>
> (Thyer, 1989: 312).

This close association between research and practice methods has fostered the development of measurement scales which can be used for both practice and research purposes. 'Rapid assessment methods' which are claimed to be short, reliable, and valid, and easy to read, to complete and understand, score and interpret, have become increasingly available (eg Corcoran and Fischer, 1987).

Efforts to widen the utilisation of empirical practice have so far met with limited success. Sheldon and MacDonald cover the reasons usually given why social workers have failed to draw on the practice consequences of effectiveness research. First, 'we are the herbalists of the helping professions. We feel we just know from personal experience which approaches work and which do not.' Second, the early evaluations were disastrous in their consequences. 'The classic recipes of a generation of textbook-writers appeared, when tried out in the kitchen, to produce either unappetising stodge or, on occasion, the social work equivalent of food poisoning.' Finally, social workers do not read much or keep up with new thinking, and employers do not encourage 'such distractions from the day-to-day work of doing good' (Sheldon and MacDonald, 1989-90: 211, 212). Probation officers, for example, have been criticised for their failure to implement effective practice, and described as 'a professional or personal preference-led service, strongly influenced by ideological positions' (MacDonald, 1994: 419-20). Hence, the responsibility for this alleged problem is laid firmly at the door of social workers, the people who employ and manage them, and 'intellectual Luddites' espousing 'so called qualitative approaches to understanding' (Thyer, 1995: 97).

What is working with offenders?

Work with offenders is the field of practice where the demand for empirical practice has gained perhaps the most attentive hearing in Britain. The policy context of probation officers' work makes the reduction of offending a continuing issue. The Home Office Research Unit gained international recognition for its research on intervention programmes with offenders in the 1960s and 1970s, through the IMPACT studies of the effects of intensive intervention with high risk offenders (Folkard *et al.*, 1974; 1976), and the work of researchers such as Martin Davies, Ken Pease and Ian Sinclair, who were subsequently to become influential within British criminology and social work education. A series of well-resourced experimental and quasi-experimental studies appeared to demonstrate that rehabilitation programmes, whether in probation teams, prison welfare units or institutions for young offenders, were 'at best...a waste of energy and commitment, and at worst...counterproductive' (Raynor and Vanstone, 1994: 398; Martinson, 1974; Brody, 1976). Subsequent attacks from political left and right provided the context for the development of a 'non-treatment paradigm' (Bottoms and McWilliams, 1979; Celnick and McWilliams, 1991) which replaced 'treatment' with 'help', informed choice, diversion, and crime prevention.

It is against this setting that the past few years have witnessed a revival of interest in treatment methods, the introduction of cognitive-behavioural methods, and the gradual rethinking of the non-treatment paradigm. Calls for accountability, the introduction of national standards for probation practice, the high profile of criminal justice legislation, and the continuing efforts of politicians and civil servants within the Home Office to distance probation practice from social work, have combined to create a political atmosphere favouring 'community strategies which offer offenders *and* our political paymasters something of value' (MacDonald, 1994: 415). Links between corrections work in Canada and Britain are not new, but they have followed a strong west to east influence with the introduction to Britain of the Reasoning and Rehabilitation programme developed by Ross and colleagues (Ross, Fabiano and Ewles, 1988). However, it is probable that the renaissance of optimism owes something at least to British work carried out in the 1980's in the intermediate treatment field (Pitts, 1992). The Ross programme argues that a focus is needed on people's *thinking*, and that offences stem in large part from offenders' failure to think actions through, and a lack of awareness of the impact of their actions on other people. An evaluation of the introduction of the Ross programme to Britain ('Straight Thinking on Probation' - STOP - in Mid Glamorgan) has been carried out. However, the interim findings are mixed, and there may prove to be few strong differences in reconviction rates between STOP group members and members of control groups (Raynor and Vanstone, 1994).

The core components of empirical practice - a behavioural focus, cognitive-behavioural methods, clear problem definition, structured objectives, and change focused intervention - are strongly in evidence within the Ross programme. But it possesses important additional features. First, the focus of work is on offence behaviour or on factors closely associated with that behaviour. 'The view that how we *relate* to clients is more important than what we *do* directly to address the "aetiology" of their and our problems is increasingly difficult to maintain' (MacDonald, 1994: 415). Second, high-risk offenders are regarded as the most appropriate target for community based intervention, and group based activities of a variety of sorts have developed vigorously. Third, the main research evidence drawn on by advocates is about individual or small group behaviour (eg McGuire, 1994), and there is a strongly pragmatic, non-theoretical readiness to capitalise on methods that appear to work. In addition, the associated research has led to the development and borrowing of a wide variety of assessment scales which can also be used within direct practice.

The main practice inference made from these developments is that probation officers should be ready to adapt their practice to the findings of research, and become effectiveness-oriented practitioners. Although this does not of itself require probation offices to turn self-evaluating practitioner researchers, there have been some spin-offs suggesting that this work with offenders may foster practitioner research. We have already noted McIvor's argument for practitioner evaluation in probation from 'the twofold belief that practitioners should be encouraged to engage in the evaluation of their own practice and that they possess many of the skills which are necessary to undertake the evaluative task' (McIvor, 1995: 210). The skills she has in mind include problem solving, effective interviewing and planning, 'which can, with a little advice and support, be readily applied in assessing the effectiveness of their work' (p217).

'What Works?' researchers have drawn partly on evidence from new research, but also on a rethinking and re-analysis of earlier evidence.   This has been based on interesting and important developments in the way in which research findings have been synthesised. The traditional method of reviewing research studies has involved a fairly intuitive interpretation of the accumulated evidence. Newer methods, called meta-analysis, involve a rigorous, non-intuitive approach to the synthesis of research findings. Designed to make disagreement among experts 'more a matter of method than opinion',

> By developing a clear set of methodological guidelines for reviewing prior research and using statistical principles to summarise the results of previous studies, meta-analysis offers the possibility of making the process of reviewing a research literature more a science than an art
>
> (Cook, Cooper, and Cordray, 1992: x).

Statistically sophisticated approaches of this kind may seem of limited interest to probation officers, and of no relevance to evaluating in practice.   Indeed, Lipsey's meta-analysis of the effects of rehabilitation for dealing with young offenders was based on 443 studies (Lipsey, 1992; 1995)!   However, the capacity of meta-analyses to take into account small effects from individual studies has proved a potent attraction. 'Meta-analyses have...generated a new source of optimism among social scientists of all types...No longer is it possible to entertain the pessimistic, simplistic and energy-sapping hypothesis that "nothing works"' (Cook, Cooper and Cordray, 1992: 14). The several meta-analyses so far completed have suggested that treatment programmes with offenders yield 'at least modest overall treatment effects' (Lipsey, 1992: 125) of about ten per cent over control groups. Deterrent and punitive programmes have been shown to lead to a marked *increase* in recidivism, and unstructured counselling approaches are said to have led to zero reductions in subsequent offending.

The case for empirical practice in work with offenders has thus gained impetus from the practice consequences of the cognitive revolution in social psychology, the technical re-analysis of previous research, and a political climate that favoured the development of an alternative to custody that was tough. The readiness of the 'What Works?' school to adjust to favourable political winds has led to some of the most cogent criticisms of these developments. Pitts claims that we have witnessed 'the replacement of a Nothing Works *doctrine* with a Something Works *doctrine*.' 'The political role of a 'Something Works' doctrine is to offer legitimacy to the government's attempts to promote an alternative, non-custodial sentencing tariff.' He complains that this has led to a professional and academic 'macho-correctionalism' and a politically prescriptive style of work, which is 'conceptually bankrupt' and will lead probation officers into a state of 'voluntary conceptual amnesia'. He fears it will do nothing to 'ameliorate the routine danger, poverty and deprivation of the lives of...young people and their victims' (Pitts, 1992). We will hear echoes of this criticism in our review of the contribution made by single-system designs.

What works with single systems?

Single subject methods in social work evaluation were initially adopted by behavioural scientists in education and psychology, who took the method from agriculture. Reports of single system evaluations have appeared in the social work literature, particularly in America, since the late 1960s (Thyer and Thyer, 1992). The strategy involves the intensive study of one client system as opposed to a more wide ranging investigation of larger groups of service users. The term 'single system (or case) *experiments*' refers to the fact that *causal* factors are being studied through *experimental* models with individual clients. 'Single system (or case) *evaluation*' refers to the use of single system designs to evaluate practice, to help identify progress, make practice decisions and as an aid to accountability. Both of these terms are part of the broader category of empirical practice, which refers, as we have seen, to using empirically tested practice methods wherever possible. The distinction between experimental and evaluation uses is emphasised by Thyer (1993: 96).

> Single system designs can be used to answer two very different types of questions, evaluative and experimental. The evaluative question is: Did the client system improve during the course of social work intervention? The experimental question is: Did the client system improve *because* of social work intervention?

The evaluative question asks whether something changed, where-as the experimental question asks whether the cause of the change can be identified. A description and explanation of single system designs are beyond the scope of this book, but are readily accessible in the literature (eg Kazdin, 1982; Thyer, 1993; Blythe, Tripodi and Briar, 1995). Roughly speaking, more simple and less intrusive designs address only the evaluative question, whereas more complex, intrusive and resource-hungry designs address both experimental and evaluative questions. All designs depend on the identification of measurable objectives, reliable and valid outcome measures, and methods of appropriately displaying the data, usually in graph form. Generally speaking, single system designs depend on processes of logical inference that identify the coincidence or otherwise of client change with specific social work intervention(s). The more complex experimental designs rely on a process of logical inference that Thyer calls 'the principle of unlikely successive coincidence' (1993: 103). If changes occur *once* in coincidence with the *introduction* or *withdrawal* of a specific intervention, then little weight should be attached to that single coincidence but if such changes occur two or more times, then that is probably too much to put down to chance. Many proponents of single system designs have grown increasingly cautious of claiming that cause and effect questions can be answered through this approach. The main criticism has been that the measurement models of single system designs are liable to distortion in the natural environment of agency practice, and the more careful commentators have concluded that 'monitoring client change should be a practitioner's primary goal, and attributing client change to the intervention, a secondary goal' (Robinson, Benson and Blythe, 1988: 298; Kagle, 1982).

Single system designs have clear attractions over more traditional group experimental designs. Apart from the obvious resource reasons for not undertaking large traditional experiments, grouped data hide the very information that individual practitioners and service users need if they are to act directly on it. For example, if a group of service users following a cognitive-behavioural programme for drink and drive offences displays better anger management skills than a group which pursued individual counselling methods, we do no know if there has been significant change in group members who started with very low anger management skills. Also, if one group is no better or worse than the other group, does this mean that none of the group members in either group has shifted, or does it mean that the members of one group are made up of some who benefited considerably and some whose skills deteriorated during the period of intervention? In other words, group measures reveal *net* change, not *gross*, individual change.   Single system designs avoid these problems.   'Unlike experimental, control group designs which compare groups, single-system designs make comparisons between time periods for the same system' (Peterson and Anderson, 1984: 12), so that the individuals act as their own 'control' over time. Advocates of single system designs believe that such methods have advantages of practical feasibility, a systematic approach, improved assessment and planning decisions, continuous feedback on performance outcomes, and, for more rigorous experimental designs, the capacity to identify cause and effect.

Challenges have been posed to more traditional counselling approaches by empirically based, systematically evaluated interventions. In the following paragraphs we will consider the relationship between helping and evaluating in these models. Are they applicable only to behavioural practice, or can they be applied to a wider cross-section of intervention methods?   Do single system designs give social workers greater certainty about practice outcomes than less apparently rigorous methods? Assuming that firm evidence about effective practice is now available, why have single system methods not met with a warmer welcome from social workers?

The new social work?

Empirical practice entails, as we have seen, a claim to 'move away from vague, unvalidated and haphazardly derived knowledge traditionally used in social work toward more systematic, rational and empirically-oriented development and use of knowledge for practice' (Fischer, 1993, p19). Its protagonists view 'research and practice as virtually the same phenomena in the clear and consistent way one views client problems, formulates hypotheses, collects information, and resolves problems' (p21). Fischer is sufficiently optimistic to prophecy the end of ideology, and to predict that 'by the year 2000, empirically-based practice - the new social work - may be the norm, or well on the way to becoming so' (p55).

Despite this optimism, there remain several important questions which have yet to be satisfactorily answered by advocates of empirical practice. *First*, it is not at all clear that empirical practice can be applied to all or even most of social work practice. Thyer argues that single system designs 'can be used in the evaluation of virtually all types of social work practice models' (Thyer, 1993: 115-

116).   Yet practice with service users whose problems are *infrequently occurring* events (eg rape or suicide attempts) is difficult to evaluate because such evaluations demand long time scales of intervention. At the opposite end of the scale, no satisfactory solution has been offered for applying empirical practice models to the high incidence of work that only involves a *single contact*. Practice that requires immediate intervention to respond to *crises*, without the space to ascertain empirical 'baselines' for problems, also poses challenges to empirical practice which have not been adequately overcome. In addition, *unpredictable* behaviour or behaviour that is part of a *complex* situation are ill-suited to single system evaluations. Almost all the examples of single system designs reported in the literature are of circumstances where the beneficiary (the client system) and the target of intervention (the target system) are the same.   Single system evaluation does not readily lend itself to practice where the intervention targets are part of the service user's wider *environment*.

Second, do empirical practice models place demands of measurement on social workers and service users which are incompatible with the realities and meaning of practice? We have seen already that promoters of the merits of 'tight' measurement in social work respond to this question with the argument that there are quantitative dimensions to all social work concepts, and therefore qualitative judgements can be translated into quantitative ones, which in turn can be counted. Some commentators go as far as to claim that 'social workers need to be numerate in order to carry out their day to day practice', and that 'numeracy is a crucial factor in the advancement of social work practice' (Taylor, 1990: 25, 30). Behavioural criteria have been favoured on the dubious grounds that 'it is possible to validate behaviour with certainty' (Fike, 1980: 48). Indeed, while no-one claims that complete certainty of knowledge can be achieved, the supporters of empirical practice believe relatively greater certainty can be gained through these methods of practice and evaluation than through qualitative methods.

Our view is that a strong base of Popper's critical fallibilism is needed.   There is no such thing as, empirical practice - only 'empirical' practice. Carol Meyer has expressed concern about such arguments on three grounds. First, she regrets the preoccupation with effectiveness defined in such a way that it can be counted, and points out that effectiveness is not the only standard against which social workers' accountability should be assessed. We pointed out in Chapter Five that ethical practice will not always be effective practice.

Second, she complains that 'most of the research methodology in use today requires the kind of narrow definition of problems and specification of variables that only behaviourist practices can provide concretely; thus it is all but impossible for practitioners who work in different modes to participate in research' (Meyer, 1984: 323). Third, she rejects the current emphasis on change as 'a new means test', and a retrograde step which abandons the understanding that social work has gained over the years regarding the relationship between individual problems and the environment.

Meyer has not been alone in asking whether empirical practice is essentially behavioural practice, and Reid has questioned whether single system designs have more than limited application in agency programmes that do not adopt highly structured interventions (Reid, 1988). Empirical practitioners have given careful attention in recent years to this question, with the result that single system designs have been applied to areas of practice much wider than cognitive and behavioural methods. Managed care, group work, psychosocial interventions, self-help methods, non-behavioural, multiple interventions with family systems, and the evaluation of social workers' practice wisdom have all been evaluated by means of single system methods (eg Corcoran and Gingerich, 1994; Fike, 1980; Jensen, 1994; Secret and Bloom, 1994; Reid, 1993; Nelson, 1993). Besa's use of a single system design to evaluate narrative family therapy demonstrates the extent to which this bridge-building has been taken. He describes an interesting piece of work that links a method based on narrative and story-telling, accomplished in collaboration with the client, with the very different traditions of empirical practice (Besa, 1994). A further example of bridge-building has been seen in the recognition by some empirical practice writers that the 'clinical mind-sets' of practitioners are important in understanding practitioner involvement in evaluation (Penka and Kirk, 1991).

The extension of single system designs to non-behavioural interventions will continue to be a central point of growth and discussion. If greater flexibility can be demonstrated for the application of empirical designs, then their attraction will spread, and the argument that such designs can be applied to everyday realities of practice will be more persuasive than it has been so far.

The debate about whether single system designs can be used for experimental purposes, to discover cause and effect relationships within practice, lies largely outside the scope of this book. Sufficient to say that there has been considerable soft-peddling on this claim in the face of serious doubts from sympathetic critics (eg Kagle, 1982;

Kazdin, 1982), and the most frequently implemented single system evaluations have been simple designs that make no claim to experimental merit (Kazi, 1994).

The *third* general question yet to be satisfactorily resolved by advocates of empirical practice is why a form of practice which places special emphasis on the provision of strong evidence for its claims should remain the method of choice of a minority of practitioners. We have noted earlier a tendency to blame social workers, agency managers and textbook writers for allowing ideology and personal preference to dictate practice rather than evidence. A more helpful response has been evident in some recent writing, suggesting that practitioner-researchers have devoted insufficient attention to the processes by which new technologies are implemented, and that they need to give greater recognition to the ethical issues raised by empirical practice.

At an early stage of this book we argued that the relationship between research and action cannot be seen simply as 'scientists understand' and then 'social workers do'. Reid describes this view of utilisation whereby findings are applied to the solution of a problem as '*instrumental utilisatio*', and argues that it does not occur very often (Reid, 1988). Probably a more common form of utilisation is '*conceptual utilisation*', in which findings are added to a storehouse of information, and emerge at some future point. We argued a similar understanding of the wider relationship between research and policy in Chapter Two. Finally, there is what Reid terms '*persuasive utilisatio*', in which evidence, ideas and understandings are used to advance a point of view. This model of research diffusion echoes discussions earlier in this book regarding rhetorical claims making and advocacy evaluation. This portrayal of utilisation processes suggests that implementation is always likely to be 'murky and convoluted' (Reid, 1988: 55). In a valuable consideration of reasons why single system designs have not been implemented by practitioners, Robinson and her colleagues underline aspects of the way in which single system evaluation, viewed as a new technology, has not undergone the ideal 'design' process. The practitioner, as the end user, has not typically been involved in design work. Also, the technology is 'not ready for implementation throughout the field' (Robinson, Benson and Blythe, 1988: 289). There are no procedural manuals and handbooks, and this hinders the use of a technology in which easy and comfortable use of single case evaluation depends on extensive experience with technical issues (p289) such as rating scales, planning a design, developing measures of baselines for problems, and interpreting data.   One reason why the Reasoning and Rehabilitation programme developed by Ross has been implemented more fully at agency level is that manuals do exist and the technology is 'user ready'.   A consequence of this weak 'design' process is that the relationship between those who develop empirical practice and those who are potential users has remained poorly developed.   The development work has been done mainly by academics, and targeted on social work students.   'Practitioners must be included in the design, refinement, and evaluation of new technologies if we expect those technologies to be implemented in practice' (Robinson *et al*, 1988: 298).

Fourthly, ethical issues have been given far too little attention. Bloom, one of the main exceptions to this criticism, has suggested the outlines of a code of ethics for evaluators in practice, in which he attempts to add the evaluative dimension to the basic Hippocratic ethics of medicine.   Hence, 'providing help' becomes 'providing demonstrable help', and 'doing no harm' becomes 'demonstrating that we do no harm' (Bloom and Orme, 1993).   He has also consistently criticised those single system designs that require the withdrawal and reinstatement of intervention (Bloom and Block, 1977).   Other questions of moral philosophy need including in the debate.   For example, it is no coincidence that Meyer should have warned enthusiasts of empirical practice against forgetting the constraints of the wider social system.   Empirical practitioners firmly reject a view of the client as socially constrained and instead emphasise human choice.   When applied to Probation practice this marks 'the renaissance of the ideology of the calculating, culpable, and hence rational, offender' (Pitts, 1992: 145).

The movement for empirical practice has brought with it important benefits.   It offers a more precise way of measuring process and progress, and educates the practitioner to expect and respond to constant feedback on performance.   It gives practitioners more control over evaluation of their own work, and may reduce inappropriate management pressure for evidence of accountability. The integration of evaluation with developments in information technology has been recognised more readily by practitioners in this tradition than elsewhere in social work (Nurius and Hudson, 1993; Mutschler and Jarayatne, 1993).   Empirical practice has also bestowed an indirect benefit on practice, in sensitising practitioners to a culture of evaluation, for example, by leading them to be more committed to defining goals, and careful about arguing from clearer evidence.   *Finally*, in a period of time when social workers are at risk of being relegated to the status of technicians, empirical practice has emphasised the expertise of practitioners.

Yet there remain serious unresolved problems.   First, anti-discriminatory practice has been almost entirely ignored by those working in this tradition.   For example, gender issues are treated simply as technical matters of bias which can be softened if not eliminated by stronger adherence to rigorous evaluative designs. Second, despite the emphasis on service users being involved in providing evaluation data, empirical practice is at root a non-participatory form of evaluating in practice.   This is due partly to its dependence on technical expertise, and in part to the ease with which empirical practice fits into an ethos of managerial control.   We have mentioned previously how a senior probation service manager was heard to conclude from the floor of a 'What Works?' conference that 'someone out there is cancelling out the good effects.   It makes me angry.   Whoever is producing those bad results has to be stopped'. Third, much of the thrust for measurement comes from within psychology.   Despite the talk of single *systems*, the *structural* dimensions of problems are largely ignored within this tradition, and it encourages a mode of intervention in which the client is treated as the target for change.   Fourth, the movement is marked by an uncomfortable mixture of pragmatism ('if it works, do it'), and a naive view that behavioural methods are value free.   The lack of immersion in the social world of practice leads to a 'patriarchal positivism' (Miller and Crabtree, 1994: 342) blind to the actual practice of social work, which involves intentions, meanings, uncertainty, intersubjectivity, values, personal knowledge and ethics.   Finally, even the most enthusiastic adherents admit that 'at this time there is no evidence that the empirically-based practitioner is more effective than the non-empirically based practitioner' (Fischer, 1993: 54).   The value of em-pirical practice to evaluating in practice will depend on how far non-behavioural applications continue to prove feasible, whether development and utilisation issues are addressed in a less arbitrary and stereotypical manner, and the extent to which the movement as a whole is marked by a greater openness to ethical issues.

Good practice on client satisfaction

'Client feedback is not a panacea.   It is one thing to be aware of a problem and another thing to be able to do something about it...Nevertheless..it provides a counterforce to the one-sided provider perspective that is prevalent in many social agencies' (Weissman, 1988: 219). We argued during Chapter Five that concentration on performance outcomes may unhelpfully reinforce such a provider perspective.   Furthermore, we recognised in Chapter Four that satisfaction with service will be low on the agenda of service users going through the criminal justice system.   Accepting these limitations, what are good evaluating in practice standards for individual social workers and teams? How should such standards be integrated within service planning and delivery, and how should they be carried out?

First, service users or their representatives should be consulted regarding how they wish their views to be canvassed. In their study of child-centred perspectives on the meaning of 'significant harm', Butler and Williamson (1994) gave children the choice as to how they would like to be interviewed - individually, in pairs, or in small groups. They held 'warm-up' sessions with the children and young people to convey this ethos, and gave them control of the tape recorder. Bond's innovative attempt to discover the views of children who were users of a family centre was organised around an imaginative activity programme (Bond, 1990-1991). Further possibilities for focus group evaluation were suggested in the previous chapter.

Second, mechanisms must be in place to take up necessary action arising from the service users' appraisal. Weissman has some constructive suggestions in this area. He argues that most agencies do not decide clearly in advance what 'point on the continuum of change they are shooting for' (Weissman, 1988: 208).   He distinguishes first order change, where the agency would not change its basic approach but would improve delivery, and second order change, where the system operating rules would be changed. Practitioner and management acceptance of client feedback will depend on believing that beneficial change is possible as a consequence. The shift of power entailed in a genuine exercise of this kind is likely to increase levels of dissent in the short term. Service users will be aware of the discrepancy between what they expect and what they receive. Practitioners will experience tension between what they are asked to do and what they believe they should do. Because of this, there should be some opportunity for practitioner feedback. Dealing with disclosure is a special issue, and one that can occur across a wide range of service users. Serious allegations may be made against social workers. The possibility needs anticipating, and procedures put in place so that the problem is not dealt with reactively.

Third, if service user satisfaction judgements are to be taken seriously, it is probably not feasible to operate a thorough pattern of evaluating in practice with every individual and family with whom the social worker comes into contact. Routine satisfaction information need to be enriched by more occasional, thorough exercises. An example of such a more thorough approach can be drawn from Fisher, Marsh and Phillips' two-phase arrangements, in which they combined an open-ended narrative from children and families with a later and more specific set of questions (1986: 22-23). More intensive satisfaction exercises should sometimes be carried out by someone who is not in a position to invoke sanctions, real or imaginary, against service users who criticise services. Although satisfaction assessments should not be limited to final outcome measures, it will sometimes be advisable to conduct such ratings at the close of service, as a means of avoiding a safe, uncritical reply. Evaluation partnerships between agencies and local centres of higher education may also provide a means of assessment that is seen to be independent and confidential, although it will continue to be the case that 'a feedback system designed with the idea of improving services for the client is not at all necessarily perceived that way by the clients themselves' (Weissman, 1988: 210).

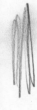

Fourth, satisfaction information is too frequently restricted to the collection of views regarding the delivery of services and perceived benefits. It should be widened to include more opportunist efforts to learn people's views about a particular problem and their opinions about the risks and benefits of introducing changes in service arrangements. In doing so, agencies and practitioners will need to decide whether they should speak to current, past or even potential service users, and whether these should be clients, carers, or advocacy groups. Feedback should be given to those who give their time to such exercises. This point is beginning to receive recognition in the special needs housing field (eg Dean, 1994; National Federation of Housing Associations, 1995).

We have concentrated mainly on the facilitating arrangements that need to be in place if service users' views are not to remain marginal tokenism. But how should the feedback be obtained? In the first place, social workers should not rely on global ratings of satisfaction. To ask a service user 'How satisfied were you with X?' is not good enough. We know from previous work that too many respondents will say they are satisfied, so the information does not allow any differentiation between service recipients or tell us what needs to be changed. Global judgements are also inadequate because expressed satisfaction is always a relative judgement - a comparison between perceived levels of problem and aspirations. Therefore, social workers must always seek to ascertain service users' aspirations and expectations. The higher the prior expectations, the more weight can be placed on the significance of high satisfaction ratings. Williams suggests that service users should be asked if they have experienced any 'bad surprises', as a way of eliciting satisfaction levels in the context of expectations (Williams, 1994). It will be helpful to distinguish between preferred (or ideal) expectations and practical ('realistic') expectations. Service users may express satisfaction if the latter are met, but their main goals will remain unsatisfied. Williams (p515) observes that a general response saying 'satisfied' may mean either

- 'I've evaluated the service and I'm happy with it', or

- 'I don't really think I have the ability to evaluate but I do have confidence in the staff', or

- 'the service was appalling but I don't like to criticise, after all they're doing their best'

The problem at this point is that the more people see themselves as powerless, the more likely they are to adjust their expectations downwards (Carr-Hill, 1992). The best practice rule of thumb is that we probably cannot obtain a meaningful picture of overall satisfaction, and should concentrate on understanding specific aspects and dimensions. The components of satisfaction in Figure 4.1 provide a general guide to the specific dimensions.

Conclusion

During this chapter we have aimed to understand the nature of the recent revival of confidence in the ability of practitioners to deliver effective interventions. We have considered the 'Something Works' assertion in the corrections field, and the growing claims for single system designs. We have concluded that there are serious shortcomings in the empirical practice movement, and that it represents an approach to evaluating in practice which is at odds with the practice model we have developed in this book. However, that criticism should not obscure the fact that the present emphasis on outcomes and measurement constitutes a challenge to practitioners which cannot be ignored.

We have returned to the research and practice that has been carried out on service user satisfaction, and recommended a good practice guide for evaluating satisfaction in practice. However, a final caution is necessary. Consumer satisfaction should not normally be regarded as an indication of practice success. 'That is tempting and unfair. It is simply too easy to make people...happy about their experience' (Fike, 1980: 46).

Throughout the book we have talked about evaluating in practice both as reflecting *in* practice and reflecting *on* practice. In the final pages we will revisit this theme, and consider whether evaluating in practice is best viewed as part of practice, or as a valuable adjunct to practice. We will consider the implications of evaluating in practice for social work education and training, and draw together the threads of our argument.

Conclusion - developing evaluating in practice

Evaluation - it's a great idea, but nobody's actually told you how.

Probation officer

Leaders of the empirical practice movement have challenged social workers and social scientists committed to humanist, participatory and qualitative methodologies to 'begin detailing just how they can actually be applied in practice' (Blythe, 1992: 268; Thyer, 1989). We have begun to do just that in the previous chapters. It has been, as we warned when we began, a mapping exercise rather than a skills handbook, in which we have worked through the outlines of an evaluating model that has occasionally been called for in the social work literature, but not, to our knowledge, attempted. The model has been translated and remodelled heavily from recent thinking and practice in the field of qualitative research methods. Accepting that an outline map is not sufficient, we have worked out 'cartoon' sketches of how such a model might work.

We have described the inevitable stance of such an evaluator - whether she be social worker or service user - as an outsider on the inside. Traditional beliefs about the relationship between evaluation and practice viewed them as two largely separate activities - different in terms of objectives, methods, and roles of those involved. Much contemporary thinking about participatory and advocacy evaluation is, as we have seen, premised on the near opposite assumption that the two are largely similar in purpose and method. The revival of confidence in empirical practice is also based to a large degree on a similar belief about the parallels between research and practice.

Our own position is different from both of these. In a very influential paper on research and service in single-case evaluation, Thomas rejected convincingly and in detail the hope that the union of science and practice could be achieved through such methods. His general argument was that the intrusion of service requirements on research design, and the intrusion of research considerations on service, combine to suggest that 'it may be a misuse of single case experimentation to employ it for purposes of service evaluation' (Thomas, 1978: 29). Although the disruption of service may in some cases be marginal, 'the threats cannot be passed off as innocuous or inconsequential. These threats pose special problems of ethics that require appropriate protections' (p28). Thomas' much quoted paper is a salutary reminder of the risks of sociological sadism to which we referred in the opening chapter. We believe that the evaluating in practice model provides substantial protection against the threat to service ethics and compromise that Thomas discusses. Yet we have made no secret of our conviction that qualitative methods are in no way exempt from ethical risks (Stacey, 1988), and that the tension of action and understanding will be ever present for both practitioners and service users who are involved in evaluating in their own cultures (Field, 1991).

Understanding evaluating in practice

There seems to be a general feeling that people would like to evaluate, and they would like to know what they are doing is effective. But nobody has told them how.

We began this book with the recognition that, in the eyes of practitioners, evaluating their own practice is a pervasive and yet troublesome aspect of their work. Troublesome in part because existing opportunities to understand and grasp the skills of evaluating - whether through social work courses, line manager supervision, or the interaction with one's peers - do not deliver the goods. Recently qualified students to whom we spoke recalled that social work courses had dealt with evaluation 'as a concept' but that it was difficult to translate into practice. The consequence was that, although social work courses drew people's attention to evaluation, 'it left me with the guilty feeling that I wasn't much better equipped to evaluate my practice.'

Practice placements do not seem to enjoy any greater success, and practice teachers admit 'it's not the bit I'm most comfortable with'. The shift in British social work education to require direct evidence of student performance has been entirely for the good, but students land in their first practice post feeling that they do not evaluate their work as they would wish. Talking of practitioners in their first job, one probation officer said, 'it's almost assumed that because they do the job they will know how to evaluate it, and they don't. That's the bottom line.'

These misgivings about social work education have been echoed by others. Brian Sheldon complained some time ago that in social work practice 'no treatment ever seems to be abandoned', and commented on the corresponding 'supermarket principle' of social work education, whereby 'students are encouraged to believe anything they like from the vast literature available to them' (Sheldon, 1978: 12). In America this usually has been viewed as a problem about the relationship between social work practice and social research, and much effort has been spent over the years on trying to get that relationship right. Several strategies have been adopted. American schools of social work first tried introducing research courses into the curriculum (Mencher, 1959). This shifted towards the production of specialist research methods literature on social work research, initiated by the early work of Norman Polansky. This led in turn to two developments. First, the effort to develop skills as research *consumers* rather than *producers*, and second, the effort to integrate practice and research teaching (Weinbach and Rubin, 1980). A different approach, the 'proper tool' strategy, grew out of a belief that assimilating and utilising research was not sufficient. The front runner in this tool kit for social workers was the single system design. Perhaps a half of social work Master's courses in America run courses on single system designs, and this has provided the foundation for efforts to 'merge partially the roles of scientist and practitioner, grounding this merger on the developing methodologies of single case evaluation' (Penka and Kirk, 1991: 513).

The general evidence, however, is that these efforts have made little impact on social work practice. For example, it seems that increased research knowledge has no discernible impact on the ability of social workers to think critically about practice (Gibbs, Gambrill, Blakemore, *et al*, 1995). Whether this is due to inadequate curriculum development, failure of agencies to provide support, or the weaknesses of the empirical practice movement, lies largely outside our concerns. The more important issue is the development of evaluating in practice competencies. However, lack of proven impact has not discouraged enthusiastic advocates from continuing to promote practitioner research and single system methods in schools of social work (Blythe, 1992).

Social work education in Britain has gone down a rather different track. Research competencies have not been required of social work students except for the occasional reference in the Central Council for Education and Training in Social Work's (CCETSW, 1995) *Rules and Requirements* to the ability to evaluate and apply tested research findings. The *Rules and Requirements* do include some useful evaluating requirements of social work students. For example, they should 'seek feedback from service users and their carers about the effectiveness, efficiency and appropriateness of the services provided, and facilitate them to make suggestions about improvements to services.' But the regulations for social work education fall short at three points. First, evaluating has not been made a core competence. Given the vagueness surrounding the meaning of evaluation, this is not good news for social work students or for practice teachers. 'Evaluation' in CCETSW requirements may mean roughly the same as 'weigh', 'understand', 'review', 'discover' or 'reflect', all of which are used in close conjunction with 'evaluate'. Second, the main statements about evaluating are not made in the context of direct practice, but in connection with working in organisations, thus confirming the association of evaluation and management. Finally, evaluation is not mentioned once in the part of the requirements dealing with social work values. A primary purpose of social work education in this field is to remove any possibility that practitioners may come to regard evaluating as only a technical matter. The present regulations do not give sufficient support to this objective.

Learning about evaluating must be integrated with placement experience. It must also be part of social work teaching about direct practice, and imaginative methods for assessing evaluating in practice, that include practice teachers, must be part of social work courses (eg Evans, Cava, Gill and Wallis, 1988).

Developing evaluating in practice also calls for changes on the part of centres of higher education. Academics working in social science research methods and social work both need to develop the 'translation' work called for throughout this book. We have said already that too few academics have shown interest in the professional and practice implications of their work (Bloor and McKeganey, 1987, 1989). There are also several circumstances in which a collaborative and consultant role between agencies, service users and social work academics would prove valuable. For instance, we suggested the potential of new developments such as focus groups and simulated clients in Chapter Eight. These will develop with more impact - both as direct evaluating methods and also as training methods - if carried out through this kind of consultancy partnership.

But the development of evaluating in practice depends on more than new learning opportunities for social workers and academics. The choice between empirical practice and evaluating in practice belongs to a wider agenda. 'In many respects the controversy about empirically-based practice mirrors the discourse about the nature and purpose of social work. Is social work primarily a technology-driven methodology, or is it a set of ideas, values and beliefs, about individuals and society?' (Witkin, 1992: 267) Our own answer is the one that Witkin himself gives. Evaluating in practice is not limited to determining whether social work is effective, but must be a means of empowerment and social change. 'By oversubscribing to the empirical model, we risk valuing effectiveness questions over moral ones, goal achievement over goal worthiness, and empirical data over personal lived experience' (p267). Evaluating in practice challenges social work to new understandings and new methodology. It recognises throughout the significance of social workers'' present evaluating-as-it-is practices. Most importantly, it holds the promise of keeping social work honest.

References

Adams, R (1990) *Self help, Social Work and Empowerment*, Macmillan.

Ahmed, S (1989) 'Research and the Black Experience' in Stein, M (ed) *Research into Practice*, British Association of Social Workers.

Altheide, D and Johnson, J (1994) 'Criteria for Assessing Interpretive Validity in Qualitative Research' in Denzin, N and Lincoln, Y (eds) *Handbook of Qualitative Research*, Sage.

Argyris, C and Schon, D (1991) 'Participatory Action Research and Action Science Compared' in Whyte, W (ed) *Participatory Action Research*, Sage.

Atkinson, D (1988) 'Research Interviews with People with Mental Handicaps' in *Mental Handicap Research,* Vol. 1, No. 1.

Atkinson, P (1990) *The Ethnographic Imagination*, Routledge.

Atkinson, P and Hammersley, M (1994) 'Ethnography and Participant Observation' in Denzin, N and Lincoln, Y (eds) *Handbook of Qualitative Research*, Sage.

Audit Commission (1986) *Making a Reality of Community Care*, HMSO.

Austin, D (1992) 'The Findings of the NIMH Task Force on Social Work Research' in *Research on Social Work Practice*, Vol. 2, No. 3.

Baker, C (1983) 'A Second Look at Interviews with Adolescents' in *Journal of Youth and Adolescence*, Vol. 12, No. 6.

Baldwin, S and Cervinskas, J (1991) *Community Participation in Research*, International Development Research Centre.

Barclay, P (1982) *Social Workers: Their Role and Tasks,* Bedford Square Press.

Barnes, M (1992) 'Beyond Satisfaction Surveys: Involving People in Research' in *Generations Review,* Vol. 2, No. 1.

Barnes, M and Wistow, G (eds) (1992) *Researching User Involvement*, Leeds University Nuffield Institute for Health Services Studies.

Barnes, M and Wistow, G (1994) 'Involving Carers in Planning and Review' in Connor, A and Black, S, (eds) *Performance, Review and Quality in Social Care*, Jessica Kingsley.

Batchelor, C, Owens, D, Read, M and Bloor, M (1994) 'Patient Satisfaction Studies: Methodology, Management and Consumer Evalua-tion' in *International Journal of Health Care Quality*, Vol. 7, No. 7.

Becker, H (1970) *Sociological Work*, Aldine.

Beresford, P (1992) 'Researching Citizen-Involvement: a Collaborative or Colonising Enterprise?' in Barnes, M and Wistow, G, (eds) *Researching User Involvement*, Leeds University Nuffield Institute for Health Services Studies.

Beresford, P and Croft, S (1993) *Citizen Involvement: a Practical Guide for Change,* Macmillan.

Besa, D (1994) 'Evaluating Narrative Family Therapy Using Single-System Research Designs' in *Research on Social Work Practice*, Vol. 4, No. 3.

Best, J (1987) 'Rhetoric in Claims Making' in *Social Problems,* Vol. 34, No. 2.

Best, J (ed) (1989) *Images of Issues: Typifying Contemporary Social Problems*, Aldine de Gruyter.

Bierman, K and Schwartz, L (1986) 'Clinical Child Interviews: Approaches and Development Considerations' in *Child and Adolescent Psycho-therapy*, Vol. 3, No. 4.

Black, T (1993) *Evaluating Social Science Research*, Sage.

Bletsas, A (1994) 'The State of Evaluation in Public Administration', European Evaluation Society Conference, Den Haag.

Bloom, M (ed) (1993) *Single-System Designs in the Social Services: Issues and Options for the 1990's*, Haworth.

Bloom, M and Block, S (1977) 'Evaluating One's Own Effectiveness and Efficiency' in *Social Work*, Vol. 22, No. 2.

Bloom, M and Orme, J (1993) 'Ethics and the Single-System Design' in Bloom, M (ed) *Single-System Designs in the Social Services: Issues and Options for the 1990's*, Haworth.

Bloor, M (1978) 'On the Routinised Nature of Work in People-Processing Agencies: the Case of Adeno-Tonsillectomy Assessments in ENT Outpatient Clinics' in Davis, A (ed) *Relationships Between Doctors and Patients*, Saxon House.

Bloor, M (1983) 'Notes on Member Validation' in Emerson, R (ed) *Contemporary Trends in Field Research*, Little Brown and Co.

Bloor, M and McKeganey, N (1987) 'Outstanding Practices: Evaluative Aspects of a Descriptive Study of Eight Therapeutic Communities', in *International Journal of Therapeutic Communities*, Vol. 8, No. 1.

Bloor, M and McKeganey, N (1989) 'Ethnography Addressing the Practitioner' in Gubrium, J and Silverman, D (eds) *The Politics of Field Research: Sociology Beyond Enlightenment*, Sage.

Blythe, B (1992) 'Should Undergraduate and Graduate Social Work Students be Taught to Conduct Empirically Based Practice? Yes!' in *Journal of Social Work Education*, Vol. 28, No. 3.

Blythe, B and Tripodi, T (1989) *Measurement in Direct Practice*, Sage.

Blythe, B, Tripodi, T and Brair, S (1995) *Direct Practice Research in Human Service Agencies*, Columbia University Press.

Bond, M (1990-1991) 'The Centre, It's for Children': Seeking Children's Views as Users of a Family Centre' in *Practice*, Vol. 7, No. 2.

Booth, D (ed) (1994) *Rethinking Social Development*, Longman.

Bottoms, A and McWilliams, W (1979) 'A Non-Treatment Paradigm for Probation Practice' in *British Journal of Social Work*, Vol. 9, No. 2.

Bowen, D (1993) 'The Delights of Learning To Apply The Life History Method To School Non-attenders' In Broad, B and Fletcher, C (eds) *Practitioner Social Work Research in Action,* Whiting and Birch.

Briar, S (1980) 'Towards the Integration of Practice and Research' in Fanshel, D (ed) *Future of Social Work Research,* National Association of Social Workers.

Briar, S and Blythe, B (1985) 'Agency Support for Evaluating Outcomes of Social Work Services' in *Administration in Social Work*, Vol. 9, No. 2.

Broad, B (1994) 'Anti-Discriminatory Practitioner Social Work Research: Some Basic Problems and Possible Remedies' in Humphries, B and Truman, C (eds) *Rethinking Social Research: Ant-Discriminatory Approaches in Research Methodology,* Avebury.

Broad, B and Fletcher, C (eds) (1993) *Practitioner Social Work Research in Action,* Whiting and Birch.

Brody, S (1976) *The Effectiveness of Sentencing*, Home Office Research Study No. 35, HMSO.

Bull, R and Shaw, I (1992) 'Constructing Causal Accounts in Social Work' in *Sociology*, Vol. 26, No. 4.

Bulmer, M (1982) *The Uses of Social Research: Social Investigation in Public Policy-Making*, Allen and Unwin.

Bulmer, M (1986) *Neighbours: the Work of Philip Abrams*, Cambridge University Press.

Bulmer, M (1987) *The Social Basis of Community Care,* Allen and Unwin.

Burchardt, N (1990) 'Stepchildren's Memories: Myth, Understanding and Forgiveness' in Samuel, R and Thompson, P, *The Myths We Live By*, Routledge.

Butler, I and Williamson, H (1994) *Children Speak: Children, Trauma and Social Work*, Longman.

Carr-Hill, R (1992) 'The Measurement of Patient Satisfaction' in *Journal of Public Health Medicine*, Vol. 14, No. 3.

Celnick, A and McWilliams, W (1991) 'Helping, Treating and Doing Good' in *Probation Journal*, Vol. 38, No. 4.

Central Council for Education and Training in Social Work (1989) *Requirements and Regulations for the Diploma in Social Work,* CCETSW.

Central Council for Education and Training in Social Work (1995) *Rules and Requirements for the Diploma in Social Work*, CCETSW.

Cervinskas, J (1991) 'Participatory Research: An Alternative Approach' in Baldwin, S and Cervinskas, J (eds) *Community Participation in Research,* International Development Research Centre.

Chambers, R (1983) *Rural Development: Putting the Last First,* Longman.

Chelimsky, E (1994) 'Where We Stand Today in the Practice of Evaluation: Some Reflections', European Evaluation Society Conference, Den Haag.

Cicourel, A (1964) *Method and Measurement in Sociology,* Free Press.

Clandinin, D and Connelly, F (1994) 'Personal Experience Methods' in Denzin, N and Lincoln, Y (eds) *Handbook of Qualitative Research*, Sage.

Clapham, D, Means, R and Munro, M (1993) 'Housing, the Life Course and Older People' in Arber, S and Evandrou (eds) *Ageing, Independence and the Life Course*, Jessica Kingsley.

Clifford, D (1994) 'Critical Life Histories: Key Anti-Oppressive Research Methods and Processes' in Humphries, B and Truman, C (eds) *Rethinking Social Research: Anti-Discriminatory Approaches in Research Methodology*, Avebury.

Cohen, A (1971) 'The Consumer's View: Retarded Mothers and the Social Services' in *Social Work Today,* Vol. 1, No. 12.

Collett, S and Hook, R (1988-89) 'Evaluating Group Care: Should We Leave it to the Experts?' in *Practice,* Vol. 5, No. 2.

Collins, P (1986) 'Learning From the Outsider Within: The Sociological Significance of Black Feminist Thought' in *Social Problems*, Vol. 33, No. 6.

Compton, B and Galaway, B (1989) *Social Work Processes,* Wadsworth.

Connelly, F and Clandinin, D (1990) 'Stories of Experience and Narrative Inquiry' in *Educational Researcher*, Vol. 19, No. 5.

Connor, A and Black, S (1994) (eds) *Performance, Review and Quality in Social Care*, Jessica Kingsley.

Conrad, K (1985) 'Promoting Quality of Care: The Role of the Compliance Director' in *Child Welfare,* Vol. 64, No. 6.

Cook, J and Fonnow, M (1990) 'Knowledge and Women's Interests: Issues of Epistemology and Methodology in Feminist Sociological Research' in Neilsen, J (ed) *Feminist Research Methods*, Westview Press.

Cook, T, Cooper, H and Cordray, D (eds) (1992) *Meta-Analysis for Explanation*, Russell Sage.

Coote, A (1994) 'Performance and Quality in Public Services' in Connor, A and Black, S, (eds) *Performance, Review and Quality in Social Care,* Jessica Kingsley.

Corbin, J and Strauss, A (1990) 'Grounded Theory Research: Procedures, Canons and Evaluative Criteria' in *Qualitative Sociology*, Vol. 13, No. 1.

Corcoran, K and Fischer, J (1987) *Measures for Clinical Practice: A Source Book*, Free Press.

Corcoran, K and Gingerich, W (1994) 'Practice Evaluation in the Context of Managed Care' in *Research on Social Work Practice*, Vol. 4, No. 3.

Corsaro, W (1985) *Friendship and Peer Culture in the Early Years*, Ablex.

Courtney, C (1989) *Morphine and Dolly Mixtures*, Honno.

Davies, B and Knapp, M (1988) *The Production of Welfare Approach*, British Journal of Social Work.

Davis, A (1992) 'Who Needs User Research? Service Users as Research Subjects or Participants' in Barnes, M and Wistow, G (eds) *Researching User Involvement*, Leeds University Nuffield Institute for Health Services Studies.

Davis, L (1985) 'Male and Female Voices in Social Work' in *Social Work*, Vol. 30, No. 2.

Dean, R (1994) 'How Good Are You?' in *Voluntary Housing*, January 1994.

Denzin, N and Lincoln, Y (eds) (1994) *Handbook of Qualitative Research*, Sage.

Denzin, N (1994) 'The Art and Politics of Interpretation' in Denzin, N and Lincoln, Y (eds) *Handbook of Qualitative Research*, Sage.

Dixon, P and Carr-Hill, R (1989) *The NHS and its Customers: Consumer Feedback Surveys*, University of York Centre for Health Economics.

Doueck, H and Bondanza, A (1990) 'Training Social Work Staff to Evaluate Practice: a Pre/Post/Then Comparison' in *Administration in Social Work* Vol. 14, No. 1.

Draper, S (1988) 'What's Going on in Everyday Explanation?' in Antaki, C (ed) *Analysing Everyday Explanation: a Casebook of Methods*, Sage.

Edwards, A and Talbot, R (1994) *The Hard-Pressed Researcher: A Research Handbook for the Caring Professions,* Longman.

Edwards, M (1989) 'The Irrelevance of Development Studies' in *Third World Quarterly*, Vol. 11, No. 1.

Edwards, M (1994) 'Rethinking Social Development: the Search for 'Relevance' 'in Booth, D (ed) *Rethinking Social Development: Theory, Practice and Research*, Longman.

Einhorn, H and Hogarth, R (1986) 'Judging Probable Cause' in *Psychological Bulletin*, Vol. 99, No. 1.

Elden, M and Chisholm, R (1993) 'Emerging Varieties of Action Research', *Human Relations*, Vol. 46, No. 2.

Elks, M and Kirkhart, K (1993) 'Evaluating Effectiveness from the Practitioner's Perspective' in *Social Work*, Vol. 38, No. 5.

Emerson, J (1970) 'Nothing Unusual is Happening' in Shibutani, T (ed) *Human Nature and Collective Behaviour*, Prentice-Hall.

Emerson, R and Pollner M (1988) 'The Use of Members' Responses to Researchers' Accounts' in *Human Organisation,* Vol, 47, No. 3.

England, H (1986) *Social Work as Art,* Allen and Unwin.

Epstein, I and Grasso, A (1992) *Research Utilisation in the Social Services*, Haworth.

Erikson, E (1959) 'The Nature of Clinical Inference' in Lerner, D (ed) *Evidence and Inference*, Free Press.

Etzioni, A (1964) *Modern Organisations*, Prentice Hall.

Evans, D, Cava H, Gill, O and Wallis, A (1988) 'Helping Students Evaluate Their Own Practice' in *Issues in Social Work Education, Vol. 8, No. 2.*

Everitt, A, Hardiker, P, Littlewood, J and Mullender, A (1992) *Applied Research for Better Practice*, Macmillan.

Field, P (1991) 'Doing Fieldwork in Your Own Culture' in Morse, J (ed) *Qualitative Nursing Research: a Contemporary Dialogue*, Sage.

Fike, D (1980) 'Evaluating Group Intervention' in *Social Work with Groups,* Vol. 3, No. 2.

Fine, G and Sandstrom, K (1988) *Knowing Children: Participant Observation with Minors*, Sage.

Fischer, J (1976) *The Effectiveness of Social Casework,* Charles C Thomas.

Fischer, J (1993) 'Empirically Based Practice: The End of Ideology?' in Bloom, M, (ed) *Single-System Designs in the Social Services: Issues and Options for the 1990's*, Haworth.

Fisher, M (ed) (1983) *Speaking of Clients*, University of Sheffield Joint Unit for Social Services Research.

Fisher, M (1992) 'Users' Experiences of Agreements in Social Care' in Barnes, M and Wistow, G (eds) *Researching User Involvement*, Nuffield Institute for Health Service Studies, University of Leeds.

Fisher, M, Marsh, P, Phillips, D with Sainsbury, E (1986) *In and Out of Care: The Experiences of Children, Parents and Social Workers,* Batsford.

Fisher, M, Newton, C and Sainsbury, E (1984) *Mental Health Social Work Observed,* Allen and Unwin.

Folkard, S, Fowles, A, McWilliams, B, McWilliams, W, Smith, D, Smith, D and Walmsley, G (1974) *IMPACT Intensive Matched Probation and After-Care Treatment, Volume I, The Design of the Probation Experiment and an Interim Evaluation*, HMSO.

Folkard, S, Smith, D and Smith D (1976) *IMPACT Intensive Matched probation and After-Care Treatment, Volume II, The Results of the Experiment,* HMSO.

Freeman, M (1993) *Rewriting the Self: History, Memory, Narrative,* Routledge.

Fuller, R and Petch, A (eds) (1995) *Practitioner Research*, Open University.

Furnham, A (1988) *Lay Theories: Everyday Understanding of Problems in the Social Sciences*, Pergamon Press.

Gibbs, L, Gambrill, E, Blakemore, J, Begun, A, Keniston, A, Peden, B and Lefcowitz, J (1995) 'A Measure of Critical Thinking About Practice' in *Research on Social Work Practice*, Vol. 5, No. 2.

Glaser, B and Strauss, A (1967) *The Discovery of Grounded Theory,* Aldine.

Goldberg, E (1970) *Helping the Aged,* Allen and Unwin.

Goode, D (1986) 'Kids, Culture and Innocents' in *Human Studies*, Vol. 9, No. 1.

Grasso, A and Epstein, I (1988) 'Management by Measurement: Organisational Dilemmas and Opportunities' in Patti, R, Poertner, J and Rapp, C, (eds) *Managing for Effectiveness in Social Welfare Organisations*, Haworth.

Greenwood, D, Whyte, W and Harkavy, I (1993) 'Participatory Action Research as a Process and as a Goal' in *Human Relations,* Vol. 46, No. 2.

Gregg-Smith, G, Jowlett, C and Morgan, J (1993) 'Jury of Your Peers' in *Community Care*, 16 September.

Guba, E and Lincoln, Y (1989) *Fourth Generation Evaluation*, Sage.

Hall, A (1974) *The Point of Entry,* Allen and Unwin.

Hammersley, M (1992) *What's Wrong With Ethnography?* Routledge.

Hammersley, M (1993) 'Research and Anti-Racism: the Case of Peter Foster and his Critics' in *British Journal of Sociology*, Vol. 44, No. 3.

Hammersley, M (1995) *The Politics of Social Research*, Sage.

Harding, S (1986) *The Science Question*, Open University Press.

Harding, S (ed) (1987) *Feminism and Methodology*, Open University Press.

Harré, R (1989) 'Language Games and Texts of Identity' in Shotter, J and Gergen, K (eds) *Texts of Identity,* Sage.

Harré, R and Secord, P (1972) *The Explanation of Social Behaviour*, Blackwell.

Hawkesworth, M (1989) 'Knowers, Knowing, Known: Feminist Theory and Claims of Truth' in *Signs: Journal of Women in Culture and Society,* Vol, 14, No. 3.

Hawtin, M, Hughes, G, Percy-Smith, J with Forman, A (1994) *Community Profiling: Auditing Social Needs*, Open University Press.

Heineman, M (1981) 'The Obsolete Scientific Imperative in Social Work Research' in *Social Service Review*, Vol. 55, No. 3.

Henderson, P, Jones, D and Thomas, D (1980) *Boundaries of Change in Community Work*, Allen and Unwin.

Henderson, P and Thomas, D (1980) *Skills in Neighbourhood Work*, Allen and Unwin.

Hepworth, D and Larsen, J (1986) *Direct Social Work Practice: Theory and Skills,* Dorsey Press.

Hochschild, A (1983) *The Managed Heart - Commercialisation of Human Feeling*, University of California Press.

Holden, G, Rosenberg, G and Weissman, A (1995) 'Gopher Accessible Resources Related to Research on Social Work Practice' in *Research on Social Work Practice,* Vol. 5, No. 2.

Hollis, M and Howe, D (1987) 'Moral Risks in Social Work' in *Journal of Applied Philosophy,* Vol. 4, No. 2.

Hollis, M and Howe, D (1990) 'Moral Risks in the Social Work Role: A Response to MacDonald' in *British Journal of Social Work*, Vol. 20, No. 6.

Holman, R (1987) 'Research From the Underside' in *British Journal of Social Work*, Vol. 17, No. 6.

Home Office (1990) *Efficiency Scrutiny of Government Funding of the Voluntary Sector,* HMSO.

Home Office (1992) *National Standards for the Supervision of Offenders in the Community*, Home Office.

Home Office (1994) *Three Year Plan for the Probation Service, 1994-1997*, Home Office.

Home Office (1995a) *National Standards for the Supervision of Offenders in the Community*, Home Office.

Home Office (1995b) *Three Year Plan for the Probation Service, 1995-1998,* Home Office.

House, E (1993) *Professional Evaluation: Social Impact and Political Consequences,* Sage.

Howe, D (1988) 'A Framework for Understanding Evaluation Research in Social Work' in *Research, Policy and Planning*, Vol. 5, No. 2.

Howe, D (1991) 'Knowledge, Power and the Shape of Social Work Practice' in Davies, M (ed) *The Sociology of Social Work*, Routledge.

Howe, D (1993) *On Being a Client*, Sage.

Hudson, W (1988) 'Measuring Client Outcomes and Their Use for Managers' in Patti, R, Poertner, J and Rapp, C (eds) *Managing for Service Effectiveness in Social Welfare Organisations,* Haworth.

Humphrey, C and Pease, K (1992) 'Effectiveness Measurement in the Probation Service: a View from the Troops' in *Howard Journal* Vol. 31, No. 2.

Humphries, B and Truman, C (eds) (1994) *Rethinking Social Research: Anti-Discriminatory Approaches in Research Methodology,* Avebury.

James, A, Brooks, T and Towell, D (1992) *Committed to Quality: Quality Assurance in Social Services Departments,* HMSO.

Jarrett, R (1993) 'Focus Group Interviewing with Low Income Minority Populations' in Morgan, D L (ed) *Successful Focus Groups: Advancing the State of the Art,* Sage.

Jensen, C (1994) 'Psychosocial Treatment of Depression in Women: Nine Single-Subject Evaluations' in *Research on Social Work Practice,* Vol. 4, No. 3.

Kagle, J (1982) 'Using Single-Subject Measures in Practice Decisions: Systematic Documentation of Distortion?' in *Arete,* Vol. 7, No. 1.

Kazdin, A (1982) *Single Case Research Designs,* Oxford University Press.

Kazi, M (1994) 'Single Case Evaluation in the Public Sector', European Evaluation Society Conference, Den Haag.

Kirkpatrick, I and Lucio, M (1995) (eds) *The Politics of Quality,* Routledge.

Kitsuse, J and Cicourel, A (1979) 'A Note on the Uses of Official Statistics' in Bynner, J and Stribley, K (eds) *Social Research: Principles and Procedures,* Longman.

Kitzinger, J (1994) 'Focus Groups: Method or Madness?' in Bolton, M (ed) *Challenge and Innovation: Methodological Advances in Social Research on HIV/AIDS,* Taylor and Francis.

Knodel, J (1993) 'The Design and Analysis of Focus Group Studies - a Practical Approach' in Morgan, D L (ed) *Successful Focus Groups,* Sage.

Kreuger, R (1994) *Focus Groups: a Practical Guide for Applied Research,* Sage.

Lakatos, I (1970) 'Falsification and the Methodology of Scientific Research Programmes' in Lakatos, I and Musgrave, A (eds) *Criticism and the Growth of Knowledge,* Cambridge University Press.

Lewis, H (1988) 'Ethics and the Managing of Service Effectiveness in Social Welfare' in Patti, R, Poertner, J and Rapp, C (eds) *Managing for Service Effectiveness in Social Welfare Organisations*, Haworth.

Lincoln, Y and Denzin, N (1994) 'The Fifth Moment' in Denzin, N and Lincoln, Y (eds) *Handbook of Qualitative Research*, Sage.

Lipsey, M (1992) 'Juvenile Delinquency Treatment: a Meta-Analytic Inquiry into the Variability of Effects' in Cook, T, Cooper, H and Cordray, D (eds) *Meta-Analysis for Explanation*, Russell Sage.

Lipsey, M (1995) 'What Do We Learn From 400 Research Studies on the Effectiveness of Treatment with Juvenile Delinquents?' in McGuire, J (ed) *What Works? - Reducing Reoffending,* Wiley.

Lofland, J (1971) *Analysing Social Settings*, Wadsworth.

Lyman, S and Scott, M (1970) *A Sociology of the Absurd*, Appleton-Century-Crofts.

MacDonald, G (1990) 'Allocating Blame in Social Work' in *British Journal of Social Work*, Vol. 20, No. 6.

MacDonald, G (1994) 'Developing Empirically-Based Practice in Prob-ation' in *British Journal of Social Work*, Vol. 24, No. 4.

MacKay, D (1987) 'Objectivity in Science' in Helm, P (ed) *Objective Knowledge: a Christian Perspective*, Inter-Varsity Press.

MacKay, D (1988) *The Open Mind*, Inter-Varsity Press.

MacPherson, I, Hunter, D and McKeganey, N (1988) 'Interviewing Elderly People: Some Problems and Challenges' in *Research, Policy and Planning*, Vol. 5, No. 2.

Mandell, N (1988) 'The Least Adult Role in Studying Children' in *Journal of Contemporary Ethnography*, Vol. 16, No. 4.

Marsden, D and Oakley, P (1990) (eds) *Evaluating Social Development Projects*, Oxfam.

Marsh, C (1982) *The Survey Method: the Contribution of Surveys to Sociological Explanation,* Allen and Unwin.

Martin, M (1994) 'Developing a Feminist Participative Research Framework' in Humphries, and Truman, (eds) *Rethinking Social Research: Anti-Discriminatory Approaches in Research Methodology,*Avebury.

Martin, R (1995) *Oral History in Social Work*, Sage.

Martinson, R (1974) 'What Works? - Questions and Answers About Prison Reform' in *The Public Interest*, Vol. 10, No. 1.

Mayer, J and Timms, N. (1970) *The Client Speaks*, Routledge.

McCracken, G (1988) *The Long Interview*, Sage.

McGuire, J (1994) 'Reviewing and Rethinking the Evidence Concerning Outcomes of Work with Offenders' Seminar Presentation to Home Office.

McGuire, J (ed) (1995) *What Works? - Reducing Reoffending*, Wiley.

McGuire, J, Broomfield, D, Robinson, C and Rowson, B (1995) 'Short Term Effects of Probation Programmes: an Evaluative Study' in *International Journal of Offender Therapy and Comparative Criminology*, Vol. 39, No. 1.

McIvor, G (1995) 'Practitioner Evaluation in Probation' in McGuire, J (ed) *What Works? - Reducing Reoffending*, Wiley.

McKeganey, N and Bloor, M (1991) 'Spotting the Invisible Man: The Influence of Male Gender on Fieldwork Relations' in *British Journal of Sociology*, Vol. 42, No. 2.

McKeganey, N, MacPherson, I and Hunter, D (1988) 'How "They" Decide: Exploring Professional Decision Making' in *Research, Policy and Planning*, Vol. 6, No. 1.

Meadows, A and Turkie, A (1988) *How are We Doing?* National Council of Voluntary Organisations.

Mencher, S (1959) *The Research Method in Social Work Education*, Council on Social Work Education.

Merton, R (1972) 'Insiders and Outsiders: A Chapter in the Sociology of Knowledge' in *American Journal of Sociology*, Vol. 78, No. 1.

Meyer, C (1984) 'Integrating Research and Practice' in *Social Work*, Vol. 29, No. 4.

Meyer, C (1992) 'Social Work Assessment: Is There an Empirical Base?' in *Research on Social Work Practice*, Vol. 2, No. 3.

Meyer, H, Borgatta, E and Jones, W (1965) *Girls at Vocational High*, Russell Sage.

Miller, W and Crabtree, B (1994) 'Clinical Research' in Denzin, N and Lincoln, Y, (eds) *Handbook of Qualitative Research*, Sage.

Morgan, D (1985) *The Family: Politics and Social Theory*, Routledge.

Morgan, D L (1988) *Focus groups as Qualitative Research*, Sage.

Morgan, D L (ed) (1993) *Successful Focus groups: Advancing the State of the Art*, Sage.

Morgan, D L and Kreuger, R (1993) 'When to Use Focus Groups and Why' in Morgan, D L (ed) *Successful Focus Groups: Advancing the State of the Art*, Sage.

Mullender, A, Everitt, A, Hardiker, P and Littlewood, J (1993-4) 'Value Issues in Research' in *Social Action*, Vol. 1, No. 4.

Mutschler, E and Jarayatne, S (1993) 'Integration of Information Technology and Single-System designs: Issues and Promises' in

Bloom, M, (ed) *Single-System Designs in the Social Services: Issues and Options for the 1990's*, Haworth.

National Consumer Council (1986) *Measuring Up*, National Consumer Council.

National Federation of Housing Associations (1995) *Good Practice Guide to Performance Information for Housing Association Tenants*, National Federation of Housing Associations.

Nelson, J (1993) 'Testing Practice Wisdom: Another Use of Single-System Research' in Bloom, M, (ed) *Single-System Designs in the Social Services: Issues and Options for the 1990's*, Haworth.

Nurius, P and Hudson, W (1993) *Human Services Practice, Evaluation and Computers*, Haworth.

Offer, J (1991) 'The Sociology of Welfare' in Davies, M (ed) *The Sociology of Social Work*, Routledge.

Olesen, V (1994) 'Feminisms and Models of Qualitative Research' in Denzin, N and Lincoln, Y (eds) *Handbook of Qualitative Research*, Sage.

Opie, I and Opie, P (1959) *The Lore and Language of Schoolchildren*, Oxford University Press.

Opie, I and Opie, P (1969) *Children's Games of Street and Playground*, Oxford University Press.

Palmer, T (1992) *The Re-Emergence of Correctional Intervention*, Sage.

Parker, W (1984) 'Interviewing Children: Problems and Promise' in *Journal of Negro Education*, Vol. 53, No. 1.

Patti, R (1988) 'Managing for Service Effectiveness in Social Welfare: Towards a Performance Model' in Patti, R, Poertner, J and Rapp, C (eds) *Managing for Service Effectiveness in Social Welfare Organisations*, Haworth.

Payne, M (1994) 'Personal Supervision in Social Work' in Connor, A and Black, S, (eds) *Performance, Review and Quality in Social Care*, Jessica Kingsley.

Pearson, G (1975) 'The Politics of Uncertainty: a Study in the Socialisation of the Social Worker' in Jones, H (ed) *Towards a New Social Work*, Routledge.

Penka, C and Kirk, S (1991) 'Practitioner Involvement in Clinical Evaluation' in *Social Work*, Vol. 36, No. 6.

Peters, T and Waterman, R (1995) *In Search of Excellence: Lessons From America's Best-Run Companies*, Harper Collins.

Peterson, K and Anderson, S (1984) 'Evaluation of Social Work Practice in Health Care Settings' in *Social Work in Health Care*, Vol. 10, No. 1.

Pfeffer, N and Coote, A (1991) *Is Quality Good for You? A Critical Review of Quality Assurance in Welfare Services,* Institute for Public Policy Research.

Philip, A, McCullough, J and Smith, N (1975) *Social Work Research and the Analysis of Social Data,* Pergamon.

Pincus, A and Minahan, A (1973) *Social Work Practice: Model and Method,* F E Peacock.

Pitcairn, K (1994) 'Exploring Ways of Giving a Voice to People with Learning Disabilities' in Humphries, B and Truman, C (eds) *Rethinking Social Research: Anti-Discriminatory Approaches in Research Methodology*, Avebury.

Pithouse, A (1987) *Social Work: The Social Organisation of an Invisible Trade*, Avebury.

Pithouse, A and Atkinson, A (1988) 'Telling the Case: Occupational Narrative in a Social Work Office' in Coupland, N (ed) *Styles of Discourse*, Croom Helm.

Pitts, J (1992) 'The End of an Era' in *Howard Journal*, Vol. 31, No. 2.

Plaut, T, Landis, S and Trevor, J (1993) 'Focus Groups and Community Mobilisation' in Morgan, D L (ed) *Successful Focus Groups: Advancing the State of the Art,* Sage.

Popper, K (1979) *Objective Knowledge,* Clarendon Press.

Popper, K (1988) 'The Allure of the Open Future' Lecture to the World Philosophy Congress.

Pratt, B and Boyden, J (eds) (1985) *The Field Directors Handbook,* Oxford University Press/Oxfam.

Rafferty, J, Glastonbury, B, Butler, I and Shaw, I (1995) *Social Work and Information Technology*, Southampton University, Centre for Human Services Technology.

Rapp, C and Poertner, J (1988) 'Moving Clients Centre Stage Through the Use of Client Outcomes' in Patti, R, Poertner, J and Rapp, C, (eds) *Managing for Service Effectiveness in Social Welfare Organisations*, Haworth.

Raynor, P, Smith, D and Vanstone, M (1994) *Effective Probation Practice*, Macmillan.

Raynor, P and Vanstone, M (1994) 'Probation Practice, Effectiveness and the Non-Treatment Paradigm' in *British Journal of Social Work*, Vol. 24. No. 4.

Reason, P (ed) (1988) *Human Inquiry in Action: Developments in New Paradigm Research,* Sage.

Reason, P (ed) (1994a) *Participation in Human Inquiry*, Sage.

Reason, P (1994b) 'Three Approaches to Participative Inquiry', in Denzin, N and Lincoln, Y (eds) *Handbook of Qualitative Research*, Sage.

Reason, P and Rowan, J (eds) (1981) *Human Inquiry: a Sourcebook of New Paradigm Research,* Wiley.

Rees, S (1974) 'No More Than Contact' in *British Journal of Social Work*, Vol. 4, No. 3.

Rees, S (1987) 'The Culture-Bound State of Evaluation' in *British Journal of Social Work*, Vol. 17, No. 6.

Rees, S and Wallace, A (1982) *Verdicts on Social Work*, Edward Arnold.

Reid, W (1988) 'Service Effectiveness and the Social Agency' in Patti, R, Poertner, J and Rapp, C, (eds) *Managing for Effectiveness in Social Welfare Organisations*, Haworth.

Reid, W (1993) 'Fitting the Single-System Design to Family Treatment' in Bloom, M, (ed) *Single-System Designs in the Social Services: Issues and Options for the 1990's,* Haworth.

Rein, M and White, S (1981) 'Knowledge for Practice' in *Social Service Review*, Vol. 55, No. 1.

Reinharz, S (1992) *Feminist Methods in Social Research,* Oxford University Press.

Richards, H and Heginbotham, C (1992) *ENQUIRE, Quality Assurance Through Observation of Service Delivery*, Kings Fund College.

Richey, C, Blythe, B and Berlin, S (1987) 'Do Social Workers Evaluate Their Practice?' in *Social Work Research and Abstracts*, Vol. 23, No. 1.

Robb, V and Hasen N (1991) *How Do We Evaluate Ourselves?* National Council of Voluntary Organisations.

Robinson, E, Benson, D and Blythe, B (1988) 'An Analysis of the Implementation of Single-Case Evaluation by Practitioners' in *Social Service Review*, Vol. 62, No. 2.

Ross, R, Fabiano, E and Ewles, C (1988) 'Reasoning and Rehabilitation' in *International Journal of Offender Therapy and Comparative Criminology*, Vol. 32, No. 1.

Rossi, P (1987) 'No Good Applied Social Research Goes Unpunished' in *Society*, Vol. 25, No. 1.

Rotheray, M (1993) 'The Positivistic Research Approach' in Grinnell, R (ed) *Social Work Research and Evaluation*, F E Peacock.

Rothschild, (1971) *The Organisation and Management of Government Research and Development*, HMSO.

Ruckdeschel, R and Farris, B (1981) 'Assessing Practice: a Critical Look at the Single-Case Design' in *Social Casework*, Vol. 62, No. 7.

Ruddock, R (1981) *Evaluation: A Consideration of Principles and Methods*, Manchester University.

Sainsbury, E (1975) *Social Work With Families*, Routledge.

Sainsbury, E, Nixon, S and Phillips, D (1982) *Social Work in Focus*, Routledge.

Samuel, R and Thompson, P (eds) (1990) *The Myths We Live By*, Routledge.

Schein, E (1987) *The Clinical Perspective in Fieldwork*, Sage.

Schon, D (1983) *The Reflective Practitioner*, Basic Books.

Schuerman, J (1987) 'Passion, Analysis and Technology' in *Social Service Review*, Vol. 61.

Schutz, A (1971) 'The Stranger: an Essay in Social Psychology' in Schutz, A, *Collected Papers, Volume Two Studies in Social Theory*, Martinus Nijhoff.

Schutz, A (1979) 'Concept and Theory Formation in the Social Sciences' in Bynner, J and Stribley, K (eds) *Social Research: Principles and Procedures*, Longman.

Scott, D (1989) 'Meaning Construction and Social Work Practice' in *Social Service Review*, Vol. 63, No. 1.

Scott, D (1990) 'Practice Wisdom: the Neglected Source of Practice Research' in *Social Work*, Vol. 35, No. 6.

Scott, J (1990) *A Matter of Record*, Polity Press.

Searight, P (1988) *Utilising Qualitative Research to Self-Evaluate Direct Practice*, Doctoral Dissertation, Saint Louis University.

Secret, M and Bloom, M (1994) 'Evaluating a Self-Help Approach to Helping a Phobic Child' in *Research on Social Work Practice*, Vol. 4, No. 3.

Seidl, F (1980) 'Making Research Relevant for Practitioners' in Fanshel, D (ed) *Future of Social Work Research*, National Association of Social Workers.

Shaw, I (1976) 'Consumer Opinion and Social Policy' in *Journal of Social Policy*, Vol. 5, No. 1.

Shaw, I (1984) 'Consumer Evaluations of the Personal Social Services' in *British Journal of Social Work*, Vol. 14, No. 3.

Shaw, I (1995) 'The Quality of Mercy: the Management of Quality in the Personal Social Services' in Kirkpatrick, I and Martinez, M (eds) *The Politics of Quality*, Routledge.

Shaw, I (1996) 'Unbroken Voices: Children, Young People and Qualitative Methods' in Butler, I and Shaw, I (eds) *A Case of Neglect?: The Sociology of Childhood*, Avebury.

Shaw, I and Al-Awwad, K (1994) 'Culture and the Indigenisation of Quality in Third World Social Research' in *Journal of Social Development in Africa*, Vol. 9, No. 1.

Sheldon, B (1978) 'Theory and Practice in Social Work: a Re-examination of a Tenuous Relationship' in *British Journal of Social Work*, Vol. 8. No. 1.

Sheldon, B (1986) 'Social Work Effectiveness Experiments: Review and Implications' in *British Journal of Social Work*, Vol. 16, No. 2.

Sheldon, B (1987) 'Implementing Findings From Effectiveness Research' in *British Journal of Social Work*, Vol. 17, No. 6.

Sheldon, B and MacDonald, G (1989-90) 'Implications for Practice of Recent Social Work Effectiveness Research' in *Practice*, Vol. 6, No. 3.

Siegert, M (1986) 'Adult Elicited Child Behaviour: The Paradox of Measuring Social Competence Through Interviewing' in Cook-Gumperz, J, Corsaro, W and Streeck, J (eds) *Children's Worlds and Children's Language*, Mouton de Gruyter.

Sinfield, A (1969) *Which Way for Social Work?* Fabian Society.

Siporin, M (1975) *Introduction to Social Work Practice*, Macmillan.

Social Services Inspectorate (1992) *Concern for Quality: First Annual Report of the Chief Inspector, Social Services Inspectorate, 1991-1992*, HMSO.

Social Services Inspectorate (1993) *Raising the Standard: Second Annual report of the Chief Inspector, Social Services Inspectorate, 1992-1993*, HMSO.

Social Services Inspectorate (1994) *Putting People First: Third Annual report of the Chief Inspector, Social Services Inspectorate, 1993-1994*, HMSO.

Social Services Inspectorate (1995) *Partners in Caring: Fourth Annual Report of the Chief Inspector, Social Services Inspectorate, 1994-1995*, HMSO.

Specht, H (1976) *The Community Development Project*, National Institute for Social Work.

Stacey, J (1988) 'Can There be a Feminist Ethnography?' in *Women's Studies International*, Vol. 11, No. 1.

Stayaert, J (1992) 'The Conflicting Needs of Social Research and Social Work' in *New Technology in the Human Services*, Vol. 6, No. 3.

Stewart, D and Shamdasani (1990) *Focus Groups: Theory and Practice*, Sage.

Strauss, A and Corbin, J (1990) *Basics of Qualitative Research: Grounded Theory Procedures and Techniques,* Sage.

Swigonski, M (1993) 'Feminist Standpoint Theory and Questions of Social Work Research' in *Affilia*, Vol. 8, No. 2.

Taylor, F (1990) 'The Numerate Social Worker' in *Journal of Social Work Education*, Vol. 26, No. 1.

Thomas, D (1975) 'The Community Worker as Stranger' in Jones, D and Mayo, M (eds) *Community Work Two,* Routledge.

Thomas, E (1978) 'Research and Service in Single-Case Experimentation: Conflicts and Choices' in *Social Work Research and Abstracts*, Vol. 14, No. 4.

Thompson, P (1978) *The Voice of the Past: Oral History,* Oxford University Press.

Thyer, B (1989) 'First Principles of Practice Research' in *British Journal of Social Work*, Vol. 19, No. 4.

Thyer, B (1993) 'Single-System Research Designs' in Grinnell, R (ed) *Social Work Research and Evaluation*, F E Peacock.

Thyer, B (1995) 'Promoting an Empiricist Agenda in the Human Services: an Ethical and Humanistic Imperative', in *Journal of Behaviour Therapy and Experimental Psychiatry*, Vol. 26, No.2.

Thyer, B and Thyer K (1992) 'Single-System Research Designs in Social Work Practice: A Bibliography From 1965 to 1990' in *Research on Social Work Practice*, Vol. 2, No. 1.

Tolman, R and Molidor, C (1994) 'A Decade of Social group Work Research: Trends in Methodology' in *Research on Social Work Practice*, Vol. 4, No. 2.

Traylen, H (1994) 'Confronting Hidden Agendas: Co-operative Inquiry with Health Visitors' in Reason, P (ed) *Participation in Human Inquiry*, Sage.

United States General Accounting Office (1988) *Program Evaluation Issues*, GAO.

United States General Accounting Office (1992a) *Program Evaluation Issues*, GAO.

United States General Accounting Office (1992b) *Health and Human Service Issues*, GAO.

United States General Accounting Office (1992c) *Housing and Community Development Issues*, GAO.

Vanheukelen, M (1994) 'The Evaluation of European Public Policies', European Evaluation Society Conference, Den Haag.

Vertere, A and Gale, A (1987) *Ecological Studies of Family Life*, Wiley.

Warren, C (1988) *Gender Issues in Field Research,* Sage.

Warwick, D (1982) 'Tearoom Trade: Means and Ends in Social Research' in Bulmer, M (ed) *Social Research Ethics*, Macmillan.

Wasoff, F and Dobash, R E (1992) 'Simulated Clients in "Natural" Settings: Constructing a Client to Study Professional Practice' in *Sociology*, Vol. 26, No. 2.

Wasoff, F and Dobash, R E (1996) *Working With the Public: Researching Bureaucrats and Professionals as They Work With People,* Avebury.

Waterhouse, L, Dobash, R P and Carnie, J (1995) *Child Sexual Abusers*, Central Research Unit, Scottish Office.

Webb, E, Campbell, D, Schwartz, R and Sechrest, L (1966) *Unobtrusive Measures: Nonreactive Research in the Social Sciences*, Rand-McNally.

Weinbach, R and Rubin, A (1980) *Teaching Social Work Research: Alternative Programs and Strategies'*, Council On Social Work Education.

Weissman, H (1988) 'Planning for Client Feedback: Content and Context' in Patti, R, Poertner, J and Rapp, C, (eds) *Managing for Service Effectiveness in Social Welfare Organisations*, Haworth.

Whitmore, E (1994) 'To Tell the Truth: Working with Oppressed Groups in Participatory Approaches to Inquiry' in Reason, P (ed) *Participation in Human Inquiry*, Sage.

Whittaker, A (1994) 'Service Evaluation by People with Learning Difficulties' in Connor, A and Black, S, (eds) *Performance, Review and Quality in Social Care*, Jessica Kingsley.

Whittaker, D and Archer, L (1990-91) 'Using Practice Research for Change' in *Social Work and Social Sciences Review,* Vol. 2, No. 1.

Whyte, W (ed) (1991) *Participatory Action Research*, Sage.

Wilding, P (1982) *Professional Power and Social Welfare,* Routledge.

Williams, B (1994) 'Patient Satisfaction: a Valid Concept?' in *Soc Science Medicine*, Vol. 38, No. 4.

Williams, R (1976) *Keywords: a Vocabulary of Culture and Society,* Fontana.

Witkin, S (1992) 'Should Empirically-Based Practice Be Taught in BSW and MSW Programs? No!' in *Journal of Social Work Education*, Vol. 28, No. 3.

Zeller, R (1993) 'Focus Group Research on Sensitive Topics - Setting the Agenda Without Setting the Agenda' in Morgan, D L (ed) *Successful Focus Groups: Advancing the State of the Art*, Sage.

Index